PROFESSIONAL WRITING IN SPEECH-LANGUAGE PATHOLOGY AND AUDIOLOGY

PROFESSIONAL WRITING IN SPEECH-LANGUAGE PATHOLOGY AND AUDIOLOGY

Robert Goldfarb, PhD
Yula Cherpelis Serpanos, PhD

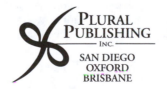

PLURAL
PUBLISHING
INC.

SAN DIEGO
OXFORD
BRISBANE

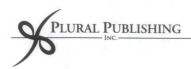

5521 Ruffin Road
San Diego, CA 92123

e-mail: info@pluralpublishing.com
Web site: http://www.pluralpublishing.com

49 Bath Street
Abingdon, Oxfordshire OX14 1EA
United Kingdom

FSC
Mixed Sources
Product group from well-managed
forests and other controlled sources

Cert no. SW-COC-002283
www.fsc.org
© 1996 Forest Stewardship Council

Typeset in 11/13 Garamond by Flanagan's Publishing Services, Inc.
Printed in the United States of America by McNaughton and Gunn, Inc.
Second printing, September 2010

Library of Congress Cataloging-in-Publication Data:

Goldfarb, Robert (Robert M.)
   Professional writing in speech-language pathology and audiology / Robert
Goldfarb and Yula Cherpelis Serpanos.
         p. ; cm.
   Includes bibliographical references and index.
   ISBN-13: 978-1-59756-175-4 (alk. paper)
   ISBN-10: 1-59756-175-4 (alk. paper)
   1. Speech therapy—Authorship. 2. Audiology—Authorship. 3. Medical
writing.   I. Serpanos, Yula Cherpelis. II. Title.
   [DNLM: 1. Writing. 2. Audiology. 3. Speech-Language Pathology.
WZ 345 G6184p 2009]
   RC423.G635 2009
   808'.066616—dc22

                                                            2009007376

CONTENTS

INTRODUCTION

"If you didn't document it, you didn't do it." Competent professional writing is a necessity, not a luxury. Third-party payers, such as insurance companies, may deny payment if the documentation for professional services is incorrect or incomplete. Medical chart notes, diagnostic evaluations, progress reports, and discharge summaries are all legal documents that may be used in court. The Code of Ethics of the American Speech-Language-Hearing Association (ASHA, 2003) states that individuals shall provide all services competently, which includes documentation of services rendered.

The authors were motivated to write the present book to address writing problems exhibited by undergraduate and graduate students in communication sciences and disorders (CSD), lax documentation by clinicians, and general slovenliness in professional discourse. In the past year, we have had our issues about professional writing shared by site visitors from the National Council for Accreditation of Teacher Education programs (NCATE), the Council of Academic Accreditation (CAA) evaluators of our graduate program in speech-language pathology, and the CAA site visitors of our consortial doctor of audiology program. In all cases, we were assured that the decline in professional writing was a national concern.

At a recent meeting of the Council of Academic Programs in Communication Sciences and Disorders, we were eager to learn how professional writing was improved in other programs. We learned that while some programs denied admission to students applying for matriculation in graduate degree programs based on poor professional writing, other programs ignored professional writing, and one was honest enough to admit, unofficially, that writing requirements were "dumbed down" to give the program a perceived competitive advantage in recruitment. All programs lamented the lack of a resource for professional writing that was comprehensive and scholarly.

In our research for the present book, we have discovered some fine style manuals for research reports and professional writing, as well as workbooks focusing on drillwork. In this volume, we hope to provide reasons and explanations for the suggestions we make, and to support our claims with relevant professional citations. We do not think our students need to attend "remedial graduate school," nor do we doubt that every CSD student and professional practitioner can learn to write competently. We also think that learning to be a better professional writer does not have to be drudgery and have attempted to leaven our instruction with humor and stories.

In Chapter 1, we describe language as our favorite toy, where even punctuation can be funny. Other topics include the alphabet soup of abbreviations that we use professionally; the mutability of language, especially among young adult users; and such thorny issues as gender neutrality and cultural differences. There are examples of correct and incorrect forms of usage throughout the first chapter, as well as exercises at the end that review some of the themes.

The focus of Chapter 2, evidence-based writing, is to provide the reader with strategies to answer the "why" questions about professional writing. While most student clinicians and professional practitioners do a fine job of explaining what they are doing and how they are doing it, there are persistent problems in differentiating science from pseudoscience and the scientific method from "common sense." We include an annotated sample of students' evidence-based writing.

As noted above, the ASHA Code of Ethics requires that we discharge our duties honorably and document our services appropriately. In Chapter 3, we review the Principles of Ethics that relate to professional writing, the constraints imposed by the Health Insurance Portability and Accountability Act of 1996 (HIPAA), and the guidelines for writing a successful research proposal to an Institutional Review Board.

As we say in Chapter 4, on using Internet resources, welcome to the new way of doing business, meeting your life partner, succeeding in academia, and conducting your clinical practice. The syntax, semantics, and jargon associated with the Internet today may appear out of date and even quaint by the time this chapter gets to the reader, but the section on uses and abuses of the Internet should remain relevant.

Using library resources, discussed in Chapter 5, begins with a history of the library, followed by a discussion of collections and services. Those of us who enjoy the musty smell of the stacks can still indulge this activity, but we also need to know how to conduct electronic searches. As the *course pack* is often used to supplement or substitute for a traditional textbook, we considered it worth noting, as well as serving as a transition to sections on copyright and plagiarism.

We have not seen a section on writing for oral presentation, which is covered in Chapter 6 in the current volume, in other professional writing books. Preparing an oral presentation is a topic of importance in basic books on rhetoric and public address, and is included here to show how to develop a speech and to outline the presentation. In delivering the oral presentation, particularly one that includes computer-generated visual aids, we differentiate what should appear on the slides compared to what should be included in effective speech delivery.

The diagnostic report, Chapter 7, is one of the lengthier sections of the book, divided into two parts. The first part specifies and describes five rules for diagnosis. For example, the second rule, *Be an Educated Consumer of Tests and Measures*, is addressed to all audiologists and speech-language pathologists, who must understand research methodology even if they do not actively produce research. The guidelines for writing diagnostic reports in speech-language pathology and audiology, in the second part of the chapter, include specific instructions and examples for diagnostic protocols and report formats.

Chapter 8, clinical reports and referrals, includes templates and samples of a treatment plan, progress report, and chart note, as well as forms of professional correspondence. We review issues in clinical writing related to terminology, ethics, and software.

We end the book with Chapter 9 on professional writing. The graduating student seeking a clinical fellowship, and the seasoned professional moving forward in a rewarding career, need strategies for developing a professional portfolio, preparing a resume, and writing a cover letter. The chapter concludes with an analysis of multiple-choice tests, those used in the Praxis II exam as well as those prepared by course instructors.

We are grateful for the assistance of Professor Suzy Lederer and Dr. Bonnie Soman in providing some of the clinic forms used in this book. Our editor at Plural Publishing, Inc., Stephanie Meissner, has provided encouragement, cheerleading, and welcome deadlines throughout the project. Our students' excellent work has inspired us, and their not-quite-so-excellent writing has motivated us, in preparing composite examples of diagnostic and treatment reports.

Neither written nor spoken words are adequate to acknowledge the support of our families. However, Shelley and Elizabeth Goldfarb deserve to know how much a sometimes preoccupied husband and father loves and appreciates them. Thanks to Andreas, Marie, and Ariana Serpanos for their unconditional love and understanding.

We invite comments and suggestions from readers to be sent to us by e-mail at:

Goldfarb2@adelphi.edu

Serpanos@adelphi.edu

RG and YCS
September 25, 2009

Reference

American Speech-Language-Hearing Association (2003). *Code of ethics.* Available from http://www.asha.org/policy

CHAPTER 1

Getting Started

Language is our favorite toy. We encourage you to play with it, develop your own skill set, and have fun inventing and reinventing your unique use of it. At the same time, we want you to develop a consistently excellent professional writing (and speaking) style, using conventions universally understood by speech-language pathologists and audiologists. The professional and personal language you use will be quite different from what the authors wrote and said as undergraduate and graduate students. Emerging technology, especially in audiology, but also in such areas of speech-language pathology as alternative and augmentative communication, has resulted in a new and richer vocabulary, with terms borrowed from computer science, engineering, and medicine.

Nowhere is the flux of language more evident than in the words used by young adults to represent something or someone in exceedingly positive terms. These have evolved from "the cat's pajamas" to "groovy," "far out," and "def." The last term gives us an opportunity to examine what is claimed here to be a misunderstanding based on vernacular English. The term *def* does not refer to hearing loss; rather, as it originated in inner cities, it refers to *death* in an ironic way. There is a phonological rule in African American Vernacular English (AAVE) where the sound made by the voiceless *th* (theta), when appearing after a vowel, is pronounced as the sound made by the letter *f*. We write the rule as follows: postvocalic /θ/→/f/. This rule, as legitimate as any other in phonology, represents the accepted practice of a large linguistic community. It is important to note the difference between vernacular English and language disorder, as Jones, Obler, Gitterman, and Goldfarb (2002) indicate in a comparison of AAVE to agrammatism in aphasia. We can see now that the use of *def* actually corresponds to a phrase—*the*

1

livin' end—used as a superlative several generations ago, for what is the end of life (*the livin' end*), but *def*?

Finally, as you play with your new language toy, resist the urge to turn nouns into verbs or verbs into nouns. Former President George W. Bush recently caused himself political harm by creating a noun from the verb *to decide*. Calling himself "the decider" resulted in a cascade of political cartoons, usually with a superhero in cape and tights (and the President's face) and a capital *D* emblazoned on his chest. The President would have been much better served by using the term *commander in chief* or even *the boss*. Similarly, creating a verb form of *clinician* is not the most apt way of expressing the notion that a speech-language pathologist or audiologist should be well rounded, as in, "To be a good clinician, you should *cliniche* with all types of cases."

BEGINNINGS OF SPEECH-LANGUAGE PATHOLOGY

This section is devoted to what we call the people we work with, and what we call ourselves. Origins of speech-language pathology are usually traced to physicians in German-speaking Europe and shortly thereafter to the University of Iowa in the United States (Goldfarb, 1985). In 1918 the University of Vienna appointed Emil Froeschels to serve as chief physician and *speech pathologist* (emphasis added) in the department of speech and voice disorders at the Central Hospital in Vienna. Together with Hugo Stern, his counterpart in the phoniatrics department, Froeschels convoked a meeting of what he dubbed the First International Congress of Logopedics and Phoniatrics. That meeting, held on July 3 to 5, 1924, at the Vienna Institute of Physiology, attracted some 65 specialists from the fields of laryngology, psychology, and pedagogical subjects. All but two of the participants were German-speaking Central Europeans.

During the 1920s the first efforts were begun in the United States to develop the study and treatment of speech and hearing problems as a nonmedical field of professional specialization. Carl Emil Seashore, a psychologist and Dean of the Graduate College at the University of Iowa, selected a promising graduate student to develop a new program. This student, Lee Edward Travis, was probably the first individual in the world to be trained at the PhD level to work experimentally and clinically with speech and hearing disorders. His preparation involved study in the departments of psychology, speech, physics, psychiatry, neurology, and otolaryngology. In 1927, Travis became the first director of the University of Iowa Speech Clinic.

At the present time the International Association of Logopedics and Phoniatrics (IALP) convenes a congress every 3 years. The American Speech-Language-Hearing Association (ASHA), which is affiliated with IALP, presently lists more than 130,000 members. The professional titles of *logopedist* and *phoniatrist* have not been adopted in the United States. (If they were, the first author of this book would have to be called a *logogerist*, because he works with the elderly.) The shift from identifying our practice as *speech correctionists* to *speech-language pathologists* is traceable to the end of World War II. When injured fighters of this war returned to Veterans Administration Hospitals (now VA *Medical Centers*) with speech and language disorders secondary to head trauma, the attending psychiatrists and psychologists found they were not equipped to deal with these communication impairments. Some psychologists, notably Jon Eisenson, acquired expertise in both psychology and speech-language pathology, but the American Speech and Hearing Association (as it was called then) began emphasizing language in the scope of practice of its members. The addition of *Language* to the title came in the 1970s, when Norma Rees was president of ASHA (which preferred to keep its acronym rather than changing it to the unwieldy ASLHA).

BEGINNINGS OF AUDIOLOGY

Audiology emerged as a distinct profession in the United States during World War II, where noise exposure to the modern weapons of the times created the necessity of diagnostic and rehabilitative services for many returning military personnel. At the time, audiologic services were administered by professionals in related areas, mostly otologists and speech-language pathologists, and included psychologists and teachers of the deaf, who ultimately became the first audiologists. The term *audiology* given to the new profession meaning "the study of (*logos:* Gr.; *audire*: L.) hearing" (Martin & Clark,

2006, p. 4) is attributed to two individuals, the otolaryngologist Norton Canfield and speech-language pathologist Raymond Carhart.

Robert West, a speech-language pathologist, is credited with expanding the discipline of speech correction to include hearing services (Bess & Humes, 2003). Audiologic services were officially recognized to be within the profession's purview by ASHA (then known as the American Academy of Speech Correction) in 1947, where the organization voted to include the term *hearing* in the association's title (Paden, 1975). At present, ASHA is the largest organization representing audiologists with over 13,000 certified members, a number that is substantially lower than the membership of over 120,000 certified speech-language pathologists also represented by ASHA (ASHA, 2008). A movement to create an independent organization for audiologists resulted in the formation of the American Academy of Audiology (AAA) in 1988 with a mission to "promote quality hearing and balance care by advancing the profession of audiology through leadership, advocacy, education, public awareness and support of research" (AAA, 2008). With over 10,000 members, the AAA is currently the largest independent professional organization operated by and for audiologists. Similar to ASHA, the AAA offers clinical certification to its qualified members, publishes a scientific journal, professional position statements, and practice guidelines in addition to consumer information, and conducts an annual national conference. There are numerous other organizations for the varying areas of audiology specializations, including hearing aid dispensing and pediatric and rehabilitative audiology.

There are physical, occupational, and respiratory therapists; why are we not speech or hearing therapists? Currently the master's degree is the minimum level of education for best practice in speech-language pathology, whereas the doctoral degree or master's level equivalent (leading to 75 credits post-baccalaureate study) is required for practice in audiology. Accordingly, speech-language pathologists and audiologists do their own diagnosis, treatment, and discharge planning. There is no medical specialty with greater expertise in communication sciences and disorders than that of ASHA-certified practitioners. Although we may provide speech, language, and aural rehabilitation, we are not therapists. A therapist's professional duties are prescribed by a physician, say, activities of daily living skills for the occupational therapist (OT) and range of motion exercises for the physical therapist (PT). Referral from a physician to a speech-language pathologist, required for some insurance reimbursement, should properly indicate no more than "evaluate and treat."

The confusion continues when we try to describe the people we treat. Those of us who work in hospitals and medical centers may refer to our *patients*. In university speech and hearing centers, our graduate students tend to see *clients*. When they go off on externships in schools, they may work with *students*. If the placement is in a day treatment center for individuals with developmental disabilities (formerly referred to as *mentally retarded*), they become *providers* working with *consumers*.

WRITING RULES

Apostrophes, Possessives, and Plurals

He who sells what isn't his'n

Must buy it back or go to prison.

(Daniel Drew, July 29, 1797–September 18, 1879)

Target Skills: apostrophes, possessives, and plurals

Most of us have been to markets where *apple's* and *orange's* are for sale. If we learn the rule that the apostrophe is used only for possession and abbreviation, but never for plurals, we will not make this mistake. We may make another mistake with possessive pronouns, though, writing *their's*, *our's*, *her's*, and especially *it's* (curiously never *hi's*; it must have to do with the placement of a vowel before the *s*), where the apostrophe should not appear. On the other hand, slavish devotion to correcting "mistakes" may interfere with our appreciation of diversity in English usage. For example, 19th-century American English included such pronouns as *your'n*, *our'n*, and *his'n*. Indeed, Drew's aphorism above works only because of the rhyme enabled by the use of *his'n*. Current usage of *dem* ("them," with the phonological rule of prevocalic /ð/→/d/) as a plural allomorph in rural areas of the West Indian island of Jamaica differs from the [s] morpheme applied to the ends of words to represent plural in urban areas of Jamaica, but is not a mistake. In a way, it may be seen as an improvement. Saying *gimme dem book* refers to a request for generic books, whereas *gimme de book dem* refers to a request for specific books.

With the *caveat* (Latin for "warning," as in *caveat emptor*, or, "Let the buyer beware") about diversity understood, some examples and exercises for apostrophes, possessives, and plurals follow. We also note that, in current professional and scholarly usage, it is no longer appropriate to use *apostrophe + s* after the name of the scientist associated with a disease. That is, *Alzheimer disease* and *Parkinson disease* are used, rather than Alzheimer's and Parkinson's. For more examples and exercises in this and other writing topics, see Hegde (2003).

Just as we exercise care to avoid using an apostrophe to turn a plural into a possessive (e.g., I bought two delicious *apple's*), we must also avoid turning a possessive into a plural (e.g., The *supervisors* desk is down the hall). Remember that the apostrophe may also be used to mark a missing letter or letters (e.g., I *can't* [cannot] do it. *That's* [that is] mine.).

1. *Evaluate the following as correct or incorrect and explain why or why not. Try adding your own examples.*

   Supervisor: Which students therapy plan is this?

   Student: Its not mine; its her's. Mine already received its grade.

The supervisor above may be referring to one or more students. If the therapy plan represented individual effort, it would be the *student's* therapy plan; if it was a group project, it would be the *students'* work. The answer by the student indicated that the therapy plan was individual work, but used an unnecessary apostrophe in the pronoun *hers*. Finally, there are different uses of the pronoun *it*. The first two uses represent an abbreviation of *it is*, and should be written as *it's*; the last usage, indicating that the therapy plan already possessed a grade, was correct. A good strategy for deciding if an apostrophe belongs with a pronoun is to use the word *is*, and then decide if an abbreviation is appropriate. In the example above, we can reasonably write, *It is not mine*, so *It's not mine* would also be correct. There is never a time that *her is* would be correct, so there can be no apostrophe in *hers*. The interaction, written correctly, follows.

> Supervisor: Which student's therapy plan is this?
>
> Student: It's not mine; it's hers. Mine already received its grade.

2. *Correct these errors*:

    1. Their's still time left to turn in your report.
    2. The toys are in the children's' playroom.
    3. How many time's do I have to remind you?
    4. They're keeping up with the Jones'.
    5. Here is a list of do's and don't's.

Corporeally Challenged

Target Skills: euphemisms, political correctness, use of adjectives as nouns

How far is too far to go in terms of political correctness? Clearly, to describe an individual as "dead" instead of the example of "corporeally challenged" used above will not offend the decedent. Should a wheelchair-borne individual see a staircase as a "physical challenge" when it is actually an impossibility?

The concept of referring to challenges stems from an important concept in rehabilitation, which is expressed as the ratio of challenge to assistance. In speech-language rehabilitation, we work to increase the client's challenge, in terms of communicative responsibility, while decreasing assistance in the form of prompts or cues. In audiology, we challenge the consumer of hearing aids to assume responsibility for maintenance and use. The philosophy is to maximize therapeutic challenge while minimizing therapeutic assistance; the more we assist, the more we have to assist, until we are figuratively killing our clients with kindness.

Euphemisms, including the family of "challenges", are created for noble reasons. We want to include people with differences, impairments, disabilities, disorders, and handicaps in the great sea of humanity; we want to focus on what makes us one, not what separates us. Accordingly, in the early 1980s, our national organization (ASHA) took a first step when it stopped using the term *aphasic* as a noun (e.g., separating *aphasics* from *controls* in experimental research) in its professional journals. The term *aphasic*, an adjective, never made much sense when used as a noun. It probably should have been *aphasiac*, to correspond with the politically (and diagnostically) incorrect use of *maniac* to describe an individual with schizoaffective disorder. We currently prefer to think of an individual who is "wearing" a disorder, rather than the other way around. We also refer to unimpaired individuals as *typical* rather than *normal*, and to individuals in experimental research as *participants* rather than *subjects*.

EXAMPLES:
Here are some examples of correct usage. Try adding some of your own.

1. Change *stutterer* to *individual who stutters*.
2. Change *autistic child* to *child with autism*.
3. Change *cleft-palate child* to *child with orofacial anomaly*.
4. Change *an apraxic* to . . .
5. Change *deaf mute* to . . .
6. Change *retarded child* to . . .

There continues to be controversy in the use of such terms as *hearing impaired* versus *hard of hearing* and *deaf*, depending on the community using the terms.

About the Deaf Community and "Hearing Impairment"

There are many terms used to describe individuals with hearing loss, including *hard of hearing* or *hearing impaired*. The use of such terms may vary depending on the severity of the loss or the communicative method used by the individual, such as manual, spoken, written forms, or their combinations. The term *deaf* is specifically used to describe an individual with a severe to profound degree of hearing loss, such that hearing cannot be used as a principal means of receiving communication. Individuals who are deaf and communicate primarily using manual language (e.g., American Sign Language, or ASL), sharing a culture of similar traditions and values, are part of what is referred to as the *Deaf community* (differentiated by the term *deaf* with a capital D). At issue with its members is the connotation of disability or handicap often associated with terms relating to hearing loss. The Deaf community does not consider deafness a deficit but rather a characteristic of an individual's hearing severity (Debonis & Donohue, 2004; Martin & Clark, 2006). In an effort to address such disparities in terminology, a position statement, *Hearing Loss: Terminology and Classification* (1998) was prepared jointly by a committee of ASHA and the Council on Education of the Deaf (CED) proposing "that terms delineating a continuum of communication function be used to describe individuals with hearing loss . . . and should reflect the personal preference of the individuals involved" (ASHA & CED, 1998. p. 22).

Our Pet, Peeve

Target Skills: punctuation, capital letters

For those whose eyes glaze over at the thought of punctuation, and cannot imagine anyone using a comma, dash, semicolon, or colon as a toy, please avail yourselves of a recording of the legendary Victor Borge performing "phonetic punctuation." You may laugh yourself off your seat.

Commas

Rules of punctuation seem to be guided by the notion that every generalization is false, including this one. Regarding commas, high school English teachers may invoke the *when in doubt, leave it out* rule, based on student compositions with commas appearing after rather than before conjunctions. Beyond the accepted convention that commas are needed between every three numbers in a group (e.g., 1,000,000 to represent one million; note the comma after *e.g.*; there would also be a comma after *i.e.*; see Latin Abbreviations below for rules on those), there are other situations where writers tend to have more trouble (Shipley, 1982).

Most references on punctuation insist on a comma before the *and* to separate items of a series of three or more (e.g., parsley, sage, rosemary, and thyme), which is called "closed punctuation." Shipley (1982) agrees, rejecting the "open punctuation" model of no comma before the *and*, and so do we.

As noted in Out-of-Control Sentences below, commas are needed in sentences with relative or nonessential clauses. However, we do not use a comma after *relative* in the sentence above, because *relative or nonessential* describes and identifies the clause. A comma is also not used between two parts of a compound predicate (e.g., *The client progressed well and was discharged from therapy.*) Finally, there is a comma after *however* (and *finally* in this sentence) when used alone to begin a phrase or sentence, but not when used as part of a phrase (e.g., *However you go, don't take the train*).

Is a comma missing? Should the comma be deleted?

1. Before you do a hearing screening make sure your audiometer is calibrated.
2. Take a case history, give the *PPVT*, and, observe attending behaviors.
3. This 68-year-old man presented with aphasia, and apraxia of speech.
4. We will use stickers and playtime as reinforcers.
5. Articulation errors consisted of substitutions, omissions and distortions of fricatives.

Answers:

1. Need comma after *screening*.
2. No comma after *and*; comma is needed after *PPVT*.
3. No comma after *aphasia*.
4. Correct; no comma needed.
5. Need comma after *omissions*.

Hyphens and Dashes

Both hyphens and dashes are made with the lower-case key to the right of the zero, one press for hyphen and two for dash. Dashes are to be used sparingly, and only when interrupting the flow of a sentence. Most sentences can be changed to avoid the use of dashes, without any obvious loss of clarity. Hyphens are used much more frequently. The *Publication Manual of the American Psychological Association* (5th ed.; American Psychological Association, 2001) notes that, with some exceptions, hyphens are sometimes used after the following prefixes:

after	intra	semi
anti	multi	sub
bi	non	super
co	over	supra
counter	post	ultra
extra	pre	un
infra	pseudo	under
inter	re	

Some words that are exceptions to the rules, and do not take a hyphen, include *bilateral, interjudge*, and *posttest*. The hyphen is always used when the same vowel is doubled, such as *re-elect,* and *co-occur*. An important qualification (Hegde, 2003) is that some words lose their hyphen and become solid words, so make sure to check current usage with an up-to-date dictionary. Finally, some compounds take the hyphen only when they precede, but not when they follow, the terms they modify (e.g., first-generation male relatives/male relatives in the first generation), or when used as an adjective, but not as a verb (follow-up activities/no need to follow up).

Colons and Semicolons

Most of us know that we use a colon before a series of items in a list, with the colon frequently preceded by the phrase, *the following*. For example, ASHA certification requires evidence of coursework in the following disciplines: biological sciences, including biology and other life sciences; physical sciences, including physics, earth science, and astronomy; social sciences, including sociology and psychology; and mathematics. Note that the items in the series of biological, physical, and social sciences are separated by semicolons, and descriptors of these items are separated by commas.

We also use colons to represent ratios, either with numerals, such as 10:1, or with words, such as male:female. For example, most authors estimate the male:female ratio of individuals who stutter as 3:1.

There remains some confusion about punctuation in notation of years and months of age in describing participants in an experiment. Generally agreed upon is the notion that a period separating years and months may be misleading. An individual who is 7 years 6 months of age is not 7.6 years; the correct notation is 7.5, because that person is 7½ years old. If it is better to avoid the confusion of the period between years and months, should there be a colon or semicolon separating them? Both have been used, with colons having more frequent use. That is, our 7½-year-old individual would be 7:6, representing 7 years and 6 months.

Finally, colons are used after the place of publication in book citations. An example, using the present publisher, is San Diego, CA: Plural.

We have seen semicolons used above, where there are items already separated by commas. Semicolons often take the place of a conjunction, when the two independent clauses are related. For example, we may write about two sets of scores with a semicolon separating the clauses instead of the conjunction *and*. Thus, *JK's bone conduction thresholds were within normal limits; his air conduction thresholds were 40 dB in the right ear.*

Semicolons are also used in referencing, using the separation by comma rule, when multiple citations are listed. For example, we might indicate that *Nursery rhymes are useful in child language development (Horner, 2006; Winkin, Blinkin, & Nod, 2007).*

Colon or Semicolon? (see Shipley, 1982, p. 54)

1. For ratios or proportions (colon, as in *10:1*)
2. Before listing a series (colon, as in, *We evaluated the following clients:*)
3. When items are already separated by commas (semicolon, as in, *ASHA conventions were held in San Diego, CA, in 2005; Miami, FL, in 2006; and Boston, MA, in 2007.*)
4. When independent clauses are not separated by a conjunction (semicolon, as in, *Our meeting will be held at 12:00; pizza will be served.*)

5. When indicating discontinuous pages (semicolon, as in *pp. 14; 23–27*)

Capitalization

Most writers are familiar with basic rules of capitalization relating to first words and proper nouns. Some, including the poet e. e. cummings and e-mail writers who insist on the lower-case *i*, seem to be making a point by flouting rules of capitalization. Frequent errors occur when capital letters are sometimes used, and sometimes not, in the same word. For example, there is a lower-case *p* in *the professor*, but a capital letter in *Professor Singh*. Another inconsistency relates to hyphenated terms. We capitalize all first letters in hyphenated titles of organizations (e.g., American Speech-Language-Hearing Association) or volumes (e.g., *Models of Short-Term Memory*), but not in titles of articles or books appearing in a reference list (e.g., *Smith, J., 2006. Noun-verb ambiguity in aging*). We also capitalize the first letter of a noun when it is followed by a numeral or a letter, such as Section 1.3 or Exhibit A. There is no universal use of the convention of using a capital letter after a colon in the title of a book or article. We agree there should be a capital *A* in such a title as, *Neurolinguistics: A book of readings*, when cited in the reference section of a journal article.

Put Your Gender in Neutral

Target Skills: s/he and [s]he; gender neutral

Most audiology students and practicing audiologists are female; the overwhelming majority in speech-language pathology is female. Some reasons for the large proportion of women in communication sciences and disorders may be the tendency to practice in schools (where the majority of teachers are female), and the ability to maintain flexible schedules in private practice and agency work, which is attractive to mothers of young children. Therefore, the default position of using the male pronoun to represent both genders seems inappropriate for our professions. Some attempts at gender neutrality in English seem natural, graceful, and effortless, whereas other formulations are awkward, clunky, and reeking of political correctness.

In many instances the efforts to avoid gender bias result in grammatical errors. Consider the following example, and try adding some of your own:

EXAMPLE:
A new graduate undertaking a clinical fellowship (CF) has questions about the ASHA Certificate of Clinical Competence. The Clinical Fellow is advised to call the toll-free ASHA hotline for clarification.

1. Standard construction, with gender bias: *When the Clinical Fellow had questions about certification, he was told to call the ASHA hotline.*
2. Politically correct, but awkward construction: *When the Clinical Fellow (Clinical Gal?) had questions about certification, she was told to call the ASHA hotline.*
3. Gender-neutral construction with grammatical error (lack of agreement between noun, *Clinical Fellow*, a singular form, and pronoun, *they*, a plural form): *When the Clinical Fellow had questions about certification, they were told to call the ASHA hotline.*
4. More graceful construction, avoiding gender, active voice: *Tell the Clinical Fellow with questions about certification to call the ASHA hotline.*
5. More graceful construction, avoiding gender, passive voice: *The Clinical Fellow with questions about certification was told to call the ASHA hotline.*

As noted above, the best way to cope with potential gender bias is to avoid using gender-specific terms. Writing *s/he* or *[s]he* is clumsy, and is not accepted in professional publications. See Battistella (1990) for guidelines for nonsexist usage.

EXAMPLE:
Avoid using s/he or [s]he by changing syntax.

1. Clumsy avoidance of gender bias: If a student arrives late to class he or she will be penalized.
2. Better construction: A student arriving late to class will be penalized.

Change these constructions:

1. A student will become a successful audiologist if s/he excels in science.
2. Everyone should accept his or her responsibilities in clinic.
3. Completing all exercises in this book will make him or her a better writer.

In a recent study comparing comprehension in nonfluent aphasia (where verbs are more impaired) and fluent aphasia (where nouns are more impaired; Goldberg & Goldfarb, 2005), one task involved ambiguous sentences. The female pronoun, *her*, was needed; the sentence could not be ambiguous with male pronouns. In the sentence, *He saw her slip on the floor*, the word *slip* could be interpreted as a noun (i.e., he saw her petticoat) or a verb (he saw her fall). However, it would take two forms of the male pronoun to make the word *crash* appear as both noun and verb.

1. She saw *him* crash at the corner (verb), and,
2. She saw *his* crash at the corner (noun).

There are times when experimental design and English syntax do not permit gender neutrality.

Gender neutrality in professional titles results in constructions which range from elegant to laughable. Some waiters and waitresses are now *waitrons, waitstaff,* or *servers.* The mailman has become the *letter carrier* or the *postal worker* (better than *mailperson, femailperson,* or *personperson*—excuse us, we're playing with our language toy again). Employment titles are an important part of an adult's case history. The following examples show gender-biased and gender-neutral occupations.

EXAMPLE:
Occupations (try adding some of your own examples).

Gender-biased	*Gender-neutral*
Steward/stewardess	Flight attendant
Policeman/policewoman	Police officer
Fireman/firewoman	Firefighter

Actor/actress	*Acter* would work, but is not used
Singer/songstress	Male version is accepted for both
Danseur/ballerina	Gender-biased foreign language terms are accepted

The final comment is an injunction for all audiologists and speech-language pathologists to earn doctoral degrees (already required for audiologists), to avoid gender bias. The doctorate is the ultimate "Ms." No one will have to decide whether or not you are to be addressed as "Mrs." or "Miss" if you are called *Doctor*. On the other hand, we recall an instructor who wrote the following on the board: *Mrs. Smith, Dr. Smith, Prof. Smith*. She said, "You may call me by any of these titles. I worked hard for all of them." Please remember that you may not be called "the doctor," which is reserved for medical practitioners.

Ye Olde Antique Shoppe

Target Skills: archaic and stilted usage; American spelling

Driving through some of the beautiful small towns of New England is an antique-lover's paradise. Some of the shops have adopted pseudo-old-fashioned spelling as a way of highlighting the antiques they sell. Unfortunately, the titles often make an unintentionally humorous mistake. The word *ye* in Ye Olde Antique Shoppe, combined with the spelling of *olde*, suggests Middle English (Remember when you read Chaucer's *Canterbury Tales*?), whereas a more recent definition of *ye* is "you". Of the many, varied, and ingenious insults created in American English, no one has ever hurled the epithet, *You old antique shop* at a transgressor. In fact, the *y* in *ye* was a variation of the thorn (/ð/, or voiced *th* sound) in Middle English, so that *ye* was pronounced as "the." The message of this anecdote is to avoid archaic usage.

American spelling does not permit the use of European English forms, such as *colour*, *centre*, and *programme*, even if Spell-Check does not highlight *centre*. European journals will accept manuscripts with American spelling, although some will change it to the forms noted above. The European notation of calendar dates is probably clearer than the American version. For example, in the section Beginnings of Speech-Language Pathology, writing the dates of the first meeting of the ICLP as 3–5 July 1924 avoids a comma, and nicely separates the days of the month from the year. However, American writers should continue to use the less clear version of July 3–5, 1924.

A decade or so ago, RG had a meeting with his daughter's first-grade teacher on Open School Night. The teacher gave a very positive report, but expressed concern about the topic of inventive spelling. It seems Elizabeth was insisting on spelling words correctly, rather than the way she thought they should be spelled, based on the way the words sounded. In an odd way, the teacher was making an interesting point. Communication through the Internet, in chat rooms, and in e-mails has resulted in a fascinating and inventive spelling system. Similarly, new terms and new forms of familiar terms seem to go through a period of natural selection where only the fittest ones survive. In the 1980s the adverbial form of the word *auditory* was written as *auditorily, auditorally,* and *auditorially*. Spell-Check doesn't have a reasonable substitution for any of these terms. The *auditorily* form seems to have survived, probably because it follows a rule (e.g., happy→happily; hungry→hungrily) accepted for other words.

Finally, professors and supervisors will not be impressed if their students use stilted vocabulary, such as *thusly* and *hence* instead of *so*, or *utilize* instead of *use*. There are places for stilted words, or they would not exist, but clinical and professional reports are generally not such places.

Are We in Agreement?

Target Skills: noun-pronoun, subject-verb, and tense agreement

Many errors of agreement represent the writer's effort to avoid gender bias by using a plural pronoun, such as *them* or *their*. Although gender neutrality is a laudable goal (see Put Your Gender in Neutral above), it is no excuse for poor grammar. The most common error of agreement is lack of correspondence between the noun and pronoun (e.g., *A student wishing to receive a change of grade must speak to their instructor first.*). The error here is lack of agreement between the singular noun, *student*, and the plural pronoun, *their*. The two easiest ways of correcting agreement are to change the subject of the sentence to a plural, (*students*), or to substitute an article for a pronoun before the object of the sentence, (*an instructor* or *the instructor*).

EXAMPLE:
Correct versions, without gender bias:

1. Students wishing to receive a change of grade must speak to their instructor first.
2. A student wishing to receive a change of grade must speak to an instructor first.
3. A student wishing to receive a change of grade must speak to the instructor first.

Subject and Verb Must Agree in Number

That is, if the subject of the sentence (which may or may not be the first noun or pronoun in the sentence) is a plural, then use the plural form of the verb. Here are some tricky examples:

EXAMPLE:

No model, whether organismic, environmental, or interactive, *is/are* adequate to explain the onset of stuttering.

Answer: *is*, because the singular form of *to be* corresponds with the singular form of *model*.

EXAMPLE:

Schuell is among the aphasiologists who *propose/proposes* a reduction-of-efficiency model.

Answer: *propose*, because the verb relates to the plural *aphasiologists*, not the singular *Schuell*.

Another Error in Agreement Involves Tense Markers

This error occurs when the writer loses control of the sentence or paragraph, usually by creating sentences that are unnecessarily complex. Consider the following:

EXAMPLE:

> *When he discussed whether or not conductive hearing loss led to delayed language development or other language disorders, Ventry shows that we must study the literature carefully.*

The agreement error in the sentence above relates to the verbs *discussed* and *led* (past tense) and *shows* (present tense). The injunction to *study* (present tense) the literature carefully does not violate agreement, even if the other verbs are past tense, because it is advice for us to take now.

Throw the Baby out the Window a Cookie

Target Skills: relative or nonessential clauses

The three sentence types—simple, compound, and complex—are well named. Not surprisingly, most writers have greatest difficulty with complex sentences. Think of a complex sentence as a simple sentence plus a relative or nonessential clause. It is fairly easy to write a simple sentence, such as, *The man ran up the stairs*, and a relative clause, such as *to catch the train*. We then have three choices. The relative clause can be right-branching, as in, *The man ran up the stairs to catch the train*, left-branching, as in, *To catch the train, the man ran up the stairs*, or center-imbedded, as in, *The man, to catch the train, ran up the stairs*. All are correct, although, in the current example, right-branching seems most natural, and center-imbedded may feel forced. The center-imbedded sentence, *Throw the baby out the window a cookie*, seems not only a forced but a criminal version of the sentence, *Throw a cookie out the window to the baby*.

Children and adults with language impairments are sensitive to increasing complexity, but so are typical language users. We can appreciate this comprehension difficulty when considering relative or nonessential clauses. In the sentence, *The cat that the dog chased jumped*, we understand that it was the dog that did the chasing and the cat that did the jumping. We can delete the word *that* and still understand the sentence: *The cat the dog chased jumped*. Theoretically, we can insert an infinite number of relative clauses into a grammatically correct sentence. However, when we insert even two relative clauses instead of one, our comprehension is severely challenged. Consider the following grammatically correct sentence: *The cat the dog the goat chased bit jumped*. The advice given many years ago by Rolnick and Hoops (1969) to use short, simple sentences when speaking to adults with aphasia certainly makes sense in this context.

Out-of-Control Sentences

Target Skills: redundancy; hyperbole; parallelism

Catching Redundancy with the Squad Squad

William Safire, the former presidential speechwriter and current columnist, deputizes his readers as members of the Squad Squad if they provide examples of redundancies. One of his deputies found three consecutive examples in a row. Get it? Writing "consecutive" makes "in a row" redundant.

Superlatives do not admit of degree. It is redundant for a merchant to describe an object as "uniquely one of a kind," because if it is unique, then by definition it is one of a kind. An infatuated boy, noting that the prettiest girl he ever saw was sipping cider through a straw, would not push his luck by describing her as the "most prettiest girl he ever saw." The rule becomes blurred when using the superlative *perfect*. The preamble to the U.S. Constitution begins, "We the People of the United States, in order to form a more perfect Union . . . "

Other terms, through accepted usage, violate the redundancy proscription with impunity. One of the more egregious of these is the part of the brain called the prefrontal area. How can an area be *pre-* (meaning "in front of") the front? Another term, used widely in advertising, is *free gift*. If it is a gift, then it is free; if it is free, then it is given away. Beware, also, of redundancies when languages are combined. Students taking winter break at *the El San Juan Hotel* in Puerto Rico probably enjoyed a *merry feliz Navidad*. Other redundant terms are found in this construction: number + "different" + varieties, kinds, or types. If a client received three kinds of language assessments, then it is redundant to write that they were "different" kinds. Hegde (2003, p. 72) has compiled a list of redundant phrases. Which word (or part) in the following phrases, appearing in our students' reports, should be deleted as redundant?

successfully completed	repeat again
precondition	hospital facilities
facilitate better comprehension	explicitly instructed
objective judges	as of yet
actual facts	in-depth analysis

Find the redundancies.

1. Three weeks following the experiment, the participants with brain damage repeated the same experiment a second time, undergoing an identical procedure.

Answer: The word "repeated" means that the participants undertook the experiment a second time. Repeating "the same experiment" means they were undergoing an identical procedure.

2. The story was presented to the participant, who was then instructed to retell the story back to the experimenter.
3. As aphasia severity increased, the patients were more impaired.

Hyperbole: "I've told you a million times, don't exaggerate."

The term *hyperbole* refers to poetic exaggeration. Most instances of hyperbole result from the clinician's inexperience. One's first client is bound to be the most fascinating, interesting, challenging, rewarding, and so on. Not that we have become jaded after more than a combined half-century of academic and clinical practice. To the contrary, we continue to be surprised by how much our students and clients teach us, and are genuinely delighted when we can make a positive impact. It is in our writing that we are less effusive.

We frequently read reports which are flowery, overwritten, and overwrought. You may note that some of the following examples contain both hyperbole and redundancy:

EXAMPLES:

1. Language and communication are two such closely inter-weaving elements as to oftentimes be virtually indistinguishable.
2. As language and communication are far from synonymous, research does well to conjecture that perhaps the collective level of communication exceeds expectations as far as the language impairment would dictate.
3. Evaluating the patients were eleven objective judges.
4. This particular study involved in-depth analysis, utilizing countless hours of videotapes, patient observations, inter-views, and videotape review.
5. Throughout the exhaustive analysis of these two patients, clinicians were targeting the use of compensatory strategies employed by the patients to combat their disability.

Parallel Lines Meet at the ASHA Convention

Imagine if Hamlet said, "To be or not being." Components of a con-struction must be matched. George Bernard Shaw's play *Pygmalion* (1916, Act II) featured the phonetician Henry Higgins (based on the English phonetics professor Henry Sweet), who was impressed by Eliza Doolittle's low-class father's use of parallelism.

> DOOLITTLE [*"most musical, most melancholy"*]: I'll tell you, Governor, if you'll only let me get a word in. I'm willing to tell you. I'm wanting to tell you. I'm waiting to tell you.

> HIGGINS: Pickering: this chap has a certain natural gift of rhet-oric. Observe the rhythm of his native woodnotes wild. "I'm willing to tell you: I'm wanting to tell you: I'm waiting to tell you." Sentimental rhetoric!

Lack of balance in pairs and series feels like the lurch of the car you drove in college; parallelism rides like a well-tuned Porche.

EXAMPLES:

> *Unbalanced:* Distractibility contributed to John's poor compliance and was a reason why his test scores were not reliable.

Parallel (balanced): Distractibility contributed to
John's poor compliance and poor test score reliability.

Be especially cognizant of correlative conjunctions, such as
either . . . or, neither . . . nor, both . . . and, and *not only* when bal-
ancing coordinate elements.

Unbalanced: Recommended follow-up is either
in-person contact at the clinic or calling him at home.

Parallel: Recommended follow-up is either in-person
contact at the clinic or telephone contact at home.

For more information on parallelism, see the chapter entitled,
"Ill-Matched Partners" (Cook, 1985, pp. 54–74).

We Saw the FLK with SOB

Target Skills: abbreviations

Not long ago, an obstetrician who noted something wrong with a
newborn would note *FLK,* for *funny-looking kid,* in the baby's
chart. This practice has, thankfully, stopped, but the avalanche of
abbreviations has not. Students and practitioners in communication sciences and disorders must become familiar with a large body
of abbreviations, and must be able to differentiate CAPD (central
auditory processing disorder) from COPD (chronic obstructive pul-
monary disease). The following non-inclusive list of abbreviations
and their meanings is an attempt to ease your study by using
groups of imaging, testing, and diagnostic abbreviations. Try adding
some of your own examples.

EXAMPLES:

Imaging (an abbreviated list)

ABR   Auditory brainstem response

CT   Computed tomography (or CAT for comput-
           erized axial tomography)

ERP   Event- (or evoke-) related potential

fMRI	Functional magnetic resonance imaging
MRI	Magnetic resonance imaging
NMR	Nuclear magnetic resonance (largely replaced by MRI)
PET	Positron emission tomography
SPECT	Single photon emission computed tomography

Testing

Tests for children (an abbreviated list)

CELF	Clinical Evaluation of Language Fundamentals
ITPA	Illinois Test of Psycholinguistic Abilities
PLS	Preschool Language Scale
PPVT	Peabody Picture Vocabulary Test

Tests for adults (an abbreviated list)

BDAE	Boston Diagnostic Aphasia Examination
MTDDA	Minnesota Test for Differential Diagnosis of Aphasia
PICA	Porch Index of Communicative Ability
WAB	Western Aphasia Battery

Diagnostic (an abbreviated list)

AD	Right ear
ADL	Activities of daily living
ASA	Aspirin
ASHD	Arteriosclerotic heart disease
AU	Both ears
Bid	Twice a day

BP	Blood pressure
CP	Cerebral palsy
CPR	Cardiopulmonary resuscitation
CSF	Cerebrospinal fluid
CVA	Cerebrovascular accident
DM	Diabetes mellitus
Dx	Diagnosis
EEG	Electroencephalogram
EKG	Electrocardiogram
EMG	Electromyogram
ETOH	Alcohol
F/U	Follow up
Fx	Fracture
GT	Gastrostomy tube
HH/HOH	Hard of hearing
HTN	Hypertension
Hz	Hertz (cycles per second)
IDDM	Insulin dependent diabetes mellitus
IM	Intramuscular
IV	Intravenous
LPN	Licensed practical nurse
LTC	Long-term care
MI	Myocardial infarction
MS	Multiple sclerosis/mental status
NGT	Nasogastric tube
NPO	Nothing by mouth

OT	Occupational therapy
PA	Physician assistant
PD	Parkinson disease
PT	Physical therapy
PVD	Peripheral vascular disease
qid	Four times a day
RN	Registered nurse
R/O	Rule out
ROM	Range of motion
SD	Seizure disorder
SNF	Skilled nursing facility
SNHL	Sensorineural hearing loss
STAT	Immediately
T	Temperature/Thoracic
V/S	Vital signs
WC (w/c)	Wheelchair
WNL	Within normal limits
X	Times
yo	Year old

By the way, SOB means *shortness of breath.*

Latin Abbreviations

In samples of students' writing, we have found considerable evidence of confusion in use of Latin abbreviations. Here are some of the most common of them.

■ The abbreviation *e.g.,* for *exempli gratia*, means "for example." If you are not sure about the use of *e.g.,* then by all means write "for example," but never write *ex-*, unless you are referring to a former partner or spouse.

■ The abbreviation *i.e.*, for *id est*, means "that is." Be careful not to use *i.e.* and *e.g.* interchangeably.

Try these exercises:

1. She needed to ace her last two exams (_____ phonetics and hearing science) to receive departmental honors.
2. The selection of courses required for the major (_____ phonetics and hearing science) was confusing.

The answer to (1) is *i.e.*, (that is), because the two choices were specified. The answer to (2) is *e.g.*, (for example), because they represented two of many choices.

Expanding an Abbreviation and Use of Plurals

Similar to the rule of plural usage (see Apostrophes, Possessives, and Plurals above), when referring to more than one item that has been abbreviated, no apostrophe is required, *e.g.*:

> Auditory brainstem responses (ABRs)

> Electroencephalograms (EEGs)

The Facts, Ma'am, Just the Facts

Target Skills: definite, specific, concrete language

One of the earliest police dramas on television was *Dragnet*, in which the detective, Sgt. Joe Friday, dealt with hysterical and evasive testimony by requesting *the facts, ma'am, just the facts*. Sgt. Friday would have had difficulty with this first sentence of an assignment to include evidence-based practice in a progress report:

EXAMPLE:

> *Extensive research studies have been conducted to determine the exact nature and extent of the*

complexity and complications involved with the impairment.

Here is another sentence that needs to go on a diet:

The first study focuses on the fact that when a word that has a stronger meaning inherent in the word or representation, the word will have a stronger impression on the memory of the patient with aphasia.

Delete the first sentence, and rephrase the second. The report now begins as follows: *Author (year) provided evidence that meaningful words improve memory in aphasia.*

Answering the Question

Following is an actual trial transcription involving the lawyer (Q), the expert witness (A), and the trial judge (The Court):

Q: Looking at Exhibits H and RR, having reviewed those documents, in your opinion was PH misdiagnosed in any way?

A: Let me first refer to Exhibit H, which is the speech-language evaluation report. There are three purposes for an initial speech-language evaluation. The first purpose is to—

The Court: No, no, please. I am in a position where if I have to try to absorb what turns out to be useless information, after a while I discard it. I am not going to be helped with a long dissertation. I would appreciate it if you would respond to the question. He asked the question as to whether or not, in your opinion, using these two documents, AB had been misdiagnosed. I would like you to answer that question first and tell me then why. Then you can expound on that in any way you wish.

The witness was evasive, because he was uncomfortable about saying a colleague misdiagnosed a patient, and was appropriately chastised by the judge for not answering the lawyer's question. Later in the transcript, a chastened witness responded to a query by the plaintiff's attorney.

> Q: I think you testified that you think BA is wrong at least to some very important elements of that evaluation, that is, her comprehension.

> A: She misdiagnosed conduction aphasia and misdiagnosed paragrammatism.

Let Me Count the Ways

Target Skills: numbers and numerals, Arabic and Roman numerals

Numbers vs. Numerals

As a general rule, write numbers below 10 as words, and numbers 10 and above as numerals. Never start a sentence with a numeral. Some applications of the rule follow.

EXAMPLES:

1. *Correct*

    There were 33 children with sensorineural hearing loss in the study.

    Incorrect

    33 children with sensorineural hearing loss participated in the study.

2. *Correct*

    I saw nine clients in the clinic today.

    Nine clients came to the clinic today.

    Incorrect

    Of the 11 clients scheduled, two didn't show up.
    (Use the numeral 2, because you are comparing it to a number 10 or above.)

Even if the number is less than 10, use numerals to represent time, date, age, as well as mathematical and statistical functions or units of measurement, e.g., Figure 3, 5%, 4 weeks, 8-channel.

Roman Numerals

Convention dictates that Roman numerals are used for cranial nerves, statistical errors, and three or more generations of males with the same name (except for royalty, which is not gender-biased, and begins with the first generation).

EXAMPLES:

1. *Correct*

   The son of John Smith is John Smith, Jr., and his son is John Smith III.

   Incorrect

   Shakespeare wrote Hamlet during the reign of Queen Elizabeth (should be *Queen Elizabeth I*).

   Queen Elizabeth, Jr. (should be *Queen Elizabeth II*) did not abdicate the throne in favor of her son, Prince Charles.

2. *Correct*

   The cricothyroid muscle is the only intrinsic muscle of the larynx innervated by the superior laryngeal nerve, a branch of Cranial X, the vagus.

   Incorrect

   There are three branches of the 5th cranial nerve (should be Cranial Nerve V or CN V).

3. *Correct*

   Assuming an effect or relationship exists when it does not is an example of a Type I error.

   Incorrect

   A type 2 error (should be Type II) accepts the null hypothesis when it should have been the rejected alternative.

Eschew Obfuscation

Target Skill: Say what the client *does*, not what the client *is*.

Consider the following interaction:

> Doctor: You are suffering from reflux esophagitis. Go to the hospital pharmacy and fill this prescription for 700 mg of calcium carbonate and 300 mg of magnesium hydroxide.
>
> Patient: Gosh, I thought I had heartburn. I was going to go to the drug store and get some Mylanta.
>
> Doctor: That's what I just said.

Why do professionals of every stripe insist on using so much professional jargon? The jaded answer is so we can charge more. Under the title of "Loose, baggy sentences," Cook (1985) skewers "officialese, prolixity, verbiage, periphrasis, windfoggery, and jargon" (pp. 1–17). However, there is improved clarity in using precise terms. A careful examination of the interaction between the doctor and patient above shows that professional terminology, properly used, yields more accurate descriptions. For example, the term *heartburn* does not refer to the heart; it is more likely a stomachache. The common use of the term *stomachache*, though, generally refers to intestinal pain. Our general rule is that the first use of a professional term that may not be universally understood should be followed by an explanatory phrase beginning with *characterized by*, or by a commonly understood synonym.

EXAMPLES:

1. *Speech-language pathology example:* JR presented with Broca's aphasia, flaccid dysarthria, and right hemiparesis.
2. Expand as follows: JR presented with Broca's aphasia, characterized by reduction of available vocabulary (especially verbs), impaired expressive syntax, and reduced speech fluency; flaccid dysarthria, characterized by reduction of speech rate, imprecise consonant formation, and hypernasality; and right hemiparesis, characterized by inability to grasp a pen to write with his dominant hand.

3. Try to expand this next example on your own: HS is currently receiving ABA 5× week for treatment of his autism.

Audiology example:

1. ST presented with bilateral otitis media, mild conductive hearing loss, and tinnitus.
2. Expand as follows: ST presented with bilateral otitis media, characterized by redness and retraction of the tympanic membranes; mild conductive hearing loss, characterized by normal bone conduction thresholds and elevated air conduction thresholds; and tinnitus, characterized by an intermittent ringing sound.
3. Try to expand this next example on your own: TH was prescribed with BTE hearing aids for his sensorineural hearing loss.

A Final Note

Here is a bit of doggerel. Consider your reaction.

With your figure asymmetrical,

Tho' you drink a case o' Metrecal,

You're a fatter man than I am,

Double Chin.

Did you notice that *tho'* really should have been written as *although* and that there really was no need to abbreviate *of* as *o'*?

Or, did you notice the play on Rudyard Kipling's rhythm, a tortured rhyme owing a debt to W. S. Gilbert (of Gilbert and Sullivan), and a tag line that rhymes with *Gunga Din*?

If you answered affirmatively to part (or all) of the first question, you'll probably make a good copyeditor, but aren't having fun with language. If you said "Yes" to part (or all) of the second question, then language is becoming your toy.

References

American Academy of Audiology. (2008). *About the academy*. Retrieved August 28, 2008, from http://www.audiology.org

American Psychological Association. (2001). *Publication manual of the American Psychological Association* (5th ed.). Washington D.C.: Author.

American Speech-Language-Hearing Association. (2008). *Highlights and trends: ASHA member counts*. Retrieved August 28, 2008, from http://www.asha.org/about/membership-certification/member-counts.htm

American Speech-Language-Hearing Association Joint Committee of the American Speech-Language-Hearing Association (ASHA) and the Council on Education of the Deaf (CED). (1998). Hearing loss: Terminology and classification; Position statement and technical report. *ASHA, 40* (Suppl. 18), 22.

Battistella, E. (1990). Language, gender, and professional writing: Theoretical approaches and guidelines for nonsexist use. *Language, 66*, 190–191.

Bess, F. H., & Humes, L. E. (2003). *Audiology: The fundamentals*. Baltimore: Lippincott Williams & Wilkins.

Cook, C. K. (1985). *Line by line: How to edit your own writing*. Boston: Houghton Mifflin.

Debonis, D. A., & Donohue, C. L. (2004*). Survey of audiology: Fundamentals for audiologists and health professionals*. Boston: Allyn & Bacon.

Goldberg, E., & Goldfarb, R. (2005). Grammatical category ambiguity in aphasia. *Brain and Language, 95*, 293–303.

Goldfarb, R. (1985). Speech disorders/communication problems. In T. Husen & T. Postlethwaite (Eds.), *International encyclopedia of education* (pp. 4760–4766). Oxford, UK: Pergamon.

Hegde, M. N. (2003). *A coursebook on scientific and professional writing for speech-language pathology* (3rd ed.). Clifton Park, NY: Thomson Delmar Learning.

Jones, J., Obler, L. K., Gitterman, M., & Goldfarb, R. (2002). The interface of phonology and morphology in agrammatism: Negation in African American vernacular English. *Brain and Language, 83*, 164–166.

Katz, J. (2002). Clinical audiology. In J. Katz (Ed.), *Handbook of clinical audiology*, (5th ed., pp. 3–8). Baltimore: Lippincott Williams & Wilkins.

Martin, F. N., & Clark, J. G. (2006). *Introduction to audiology* (9th ed.). Boston: Allyn & Bacon.

Paden, E. P. (1975). ASHA in retrospect: Fiftieth anniversary reflections. *ASHA, 17*(9), 571–572.

Rolnick, M., & Hoops, M. (1969). Aphasia as seen by the aphasic. *Journal of Speech and Hearing Disorders, 34*, 48–53.

Shipley, K. G. (Ed.). (1982). *A style guide for writers in communicative disorders*. Tucson, AZ: Communication Skill Builders.

EXERCISES

Find and correct the errors, or recast the sentence.

1. The book's are Joans, not her's.

2. John was phonically challenged after his partial laryngectomy.

3. As a member of the deaf community, Bill hoped his new baby would be born Deaf.

4. The complete package includes hearing aid, case and batteries.

5. The diagnosis was Asperger's syndrome, a mild form of Autism.

6. If s/he wants a 2:00 appointment, try to give it to him/her.

7. You may extract a biscuit from the tin if you name the correct colour.

8. A child has a right to express their own opinion.

9. At the beginning of therapy, Mary presented with a voice quality that sounds breathy.

10. Goals were met, because he answered correctly three times in a row, consecutively.

11. He made fantastic progress in therapy.

12. She improved in reading, writing, and ability to produce gestures.

13. Jim was treated for speech problems related to CP.

14. Linda can produce some consonant clusters, but not others.

15. John was tested on Form a of the *Peabody Picture Vocabulary Test,* IInd edition.

16. Mike has expressive aphasia.

ANSWERS

1. There are three errors, all involving the use of the apostrophe. A plural noun (*books*) does not require an apostrophe before the *s*; a proper noun (*Joan's*) needs an apostrophe before the *s* to represent possessive; and a pronoun (*hers*) does not take an apostrophe. The sentence should be written as follows: The books are Joan's, not hers.

2. The euphemism, *phonically challenged*, is not useful, and should not substitute for a clearer description, such as the following: John was unable to produce adequate vocal pitch and volume after his partial laryngectomy.

3. Use a capital letter to represent the Deaf community, and the lower-case form to describe profound hearing loss. As a member of the Deaf community, Bill hoped his new baby would be born deaf.

4. Use a comma after nouns in a series. The complete package includes hearing aid, case, and batteries.

5. We use an upper-case first letter when a disorder is named after an individual, but do not use a capital letter for a disorder which is not also a proper name. The diagnosis was Asperger's syndrome, a mild form of autism.

6. The attempt at gender neutrality resulted in an awkward sentence. Maintain gender neutrality by recasting the sentence as follows: Try to accommodate the client's request for a specific appointment time.

7. Avoid stilted language and use American spelling, as follows: You may take a cookie if you name the correct color.

8. The plural pronoun (*their*) does not agree with the singular noun (*child*); this was an attempt to maintain gender neutrality by avoiding the use of *his* or *her*. There are many

alternative ways of recasting the sentence; here is one: A child has a right to a personal opinion.

9. The tenses of the verbs, *presented* and *sounds*, do not agree. Use past tense for both verbs, as follows: At the beginning of therapy, Mary presented with a voice quality that sounded breathy.

10. Avoid redundancy by deleting the word *consecutively*, which is already specified by the phrase *in a row*.

11. Avoid hyperbole by changing the word *fantastic* to excellent.

12. The sentence lacks parallelism. Change as follows: She improved in reading, writing, and gesturing.

13. The abbreviation *CP* may refer to cleft palate or cerebral palsy. Avoid abbreviations in the first usage of professional terms, unless they are universally understood.

14. The description of the articulation errors is too general. Indicate the specific consonant clusters mastered and those that should be the target of future therapy.

15. Use an upper-case letter to indicate which form was used, and Arabic numbers, not Roman numerals, to indicate the edition of a test, as follows: John was tested on Form A of the *Peabody Picture Vocabulary Test, 2nd edition*.

16. The term, *expressive aphasia*, is not an appropriate professional term, because aphasia is a disorder which crosses all language modalities. In addition, it is always better to write what the client does, not merely what the client has.

CHAPTER 2

Evidence-Based Writing

The practices of speech-language pathology and audiology, as scientific professions, rely on two assurances to the public (Finn, Bothe, & Bramlett, 2005):

1. We derive and base our conclusions about communication disorders on scientific evidence.
2. Assessment and treatment are evaluated by empirical methods.

Following is ASHA's position statement on evidence-based practice in communication disorders (American Speech-Language-Hearing Association [ASHA], 2005, reprinted with permission):

> It is the position of the American Speech-Language-Hearing Association that audiologists and speech-language pathologists incorporate the principles of evidence-based practice in clinical decision making to provide high quality clinical care. The term *evidence-based practice* refers to an approach in which current, high-quality research evidence is integrated with practitioner expertise and client preferences and values into the process of making clinical decisions. In making clinical practice evidence-based, audiologists and speech-language pathologists:
>
> 1. recognize the needs, abilities, values, preferences, and interests of individuals and families to whom they provide clinical services, and integrate those factors along with best current research evidence and their clinical expertise in making clinical decisions;
> 2. acquire and maintain the knowledge and skills that are necessary to provide high quality professional services, including knowledge and skills related to evidence-based practice;

3. evaluate prevention, screening, and diagnostic procedures, protocols, and measures to identify maximally informative and cost-effective diagnostic and screening tools, using recognized appraisal criteria described in the evidence-based practice literature;

4. evaluate the efficacy, effectiveness, and efficiency of clinical protocols for prevention, treatment, and enhancement using criteria recognized in the evidence-based practice literature;

5. evaluate the quality of evidence appearing in any source or format, including journal articles, textbooks, continuing education offerings, newsletters, advertising, and Web-based products, prior to incorporating such evidence into clinical decision making; and

6. monitor and incorporate new and high quality research evidence having implications for clinical practice.

This chapter begins with a description of the scientific method, followed by a comparison of the scientific method to "common sense" and pseudoscience. The last portion will be an analysis of student written work for adherence to the scientific method in reporting.

The Scientific Method

The rules of science describe and explain phenomena, and are different from those of magic, the pseudosciences, and common sense. Anderson (1971) proposes five rules, four for description and one for explanation, unique to the scientific method.

Empirical Verification

Descriptive statements must correspond with observed reality. We define *observed reality* as sense data (which rules out intuition and divine revelation) on which different observers agree (which rules out hallucinations). As others may do the observing for us, there are rules for reporting:

■ Specific operations are required for making the observations.
■ Observations are reported.

- There is clear reasoning that leads from observations to statements.
- The process is described clearly and in sufficient detail for us to evaluate it.
- The authority of the person making the statement should be irrelevant.

The other three rules for description are specific procedures for empirical verification.

Operational Definition

All terms in a descriptive statement are defined by the operations involved in manipulating or observing their referents. For example, we want to test the following:

> Patients who *benefit* most from group treatment have been assessed as having:
>
> _____ mild aphasia   _____ moderate aphasia
> _____ severe aphasia

If "benefit" refers to improved naming and word finding, the answer might be "mild aphasia." If "benefit" refers to improved social interactions and quality of life, the answer might be "severe aphasia."

An operational definition is like a recipe: it is a set of instructions. The truth of the statement, "Julia Child liked Boston cream pie," depended on the recipe.

Schuell, Jenkins, and Jimenez-Pabon (1964) wrote that what you do about aphasia depends on what you think aphasia is. An operational definition requires that we specify what we are talking about in the following ways:

- We use only sense data in descriptive statements.
- Our meaning is clear enough that different observers can agree on the sense data.

If we have succeeded, our operational definition is a testable statement. That means it can be falsified or strengthened, but not proven.

Controlled Observation

If a change in condition or event A causes a change in condition or event B, then:

1. B must be observed when there are different values of A; and
2. all variables other than A are discounted as causes of the change observed in B.

Compare the above with the *post hoc* fallacy described in Uncontrolled Observation below.

Consider this advertisement: "The next time you service your hearing aids, replace your present batteries with Bob's batteries, and you'll be amazed at the difference." It would be amazing if there were not a difference. The kind of battery is not the only variable that could produce a change in performance. Others include:

1. condition of the present batteries;
2. condition of the hearing aids before servicing;
3. switching to Bob's; and
4. some combination of these factors.

There are five bases for discounting one variable as a possible cause of an observed change on another, as the following sections explain.

Experimental Control

Keep variables constant so that the same value occurs at each value on variable A. By using only new hearing aids and only new batteries, perfect running order (the same value of this variable) will occur at each of the two values of variable A, Bob's and Brand X batteries. Variables that do not change cannot produce changes on any other variable.

Statistical Control

Estimate the magnitude of the effect the variable will have on variable B and subtract this from the change that is observed. If removing cerumen lowers threshold by 10 dB, then we add 10 dB to thresholds after both removing cerumen and installing Bob's batteries. Whatever difference remains can be attributed to the change caused by Bob's batteries.

Assuming Invariance

You neither control nor measure the variable in question, but assume that it does not vary appreciably. Humidity affects comfort level, possibly reducing performance. If hearing aid batteries are tested one right after the other, then any change in humidity would probably be so slight as to be negligible.

Assuming Irrelevance

You don't care at all whether the same value of the variable occurs at each value of variable A. You assume that the variable has no effect on variable B. The color of the hearing aid is such a variable; you wouldn't bother to match the aids on color, because color is irrelevant to performance.

Randomization

Manipulate the variable in a strictly random fashion with respect to variable A, so that the same average value will be likely to occur at each value on variable A. Test a large number of hearing aid users, and toss a coin to decide whether to install Bob's or Brand X batteries.

Statistical Generalization

It is impossible to observe every individual or condition representing the communication disorder we wish to study. One way we use statistics is to test a random sample of individuals with a certain condition (say, 30 adults with Broca's aphasia) and generalize the findings to a larger population (all adults with Broca's aphasia). We may also want to generalize an observation to other conditions, which is an important part of carryover exercises in therapy. For example, it is important to generalize the child's language gains made in the clinic to home and school environments. The way to accomplish these goals is to obtain random samples from the set of conditions or set of individuals.

Statistical inference is the procedure for deciding if the size of the effect and the number of participants justify generalizing the result from the sample to the population. For many of the analyses we do in research, the statistical difference between 30 samples and infinity samples is trivial. Obtaining 30 samples is usually sufficient to limit the effect of small number error.

Empirical Confirmation

An explanatory statement is more likely to be true when it is consistent with:

1. verified descriptive statements and
2. confirmed explanatory statements.

Inconsistency between a descriptive statement and an explanatory statement leads to rejection of the explanatory statement.

Using the principle of controlled observation, we may propose the following:

If A, then B

Not B

Therefore, not A

Or,

If it is raining (A), the streets will be wet (B).

The streets are not wet (not B).

Therefore, it is not raining (not A).

However, one successful prediction is not sufficient to prove the explanatory statement that logically implies it, nor are two, nor, in most cases, are 100. Based on the fact that the streets are wet, we cannot be certain that it is raining (it could be the result of open fire hydrants). Successful predictions confirm the explanatory statement, or increase the probability of its being correct.

The term *hypothesis* is used to refer to a statement, either descriptive or, as in this case, explanatory, that has not yet been adequately tested. A clinical hypothesis, such as the following type, proposed by Santo Pietro and Goldfarb (1995, p. 8), is written to test the efficacy of descriptive or explanatory statements used in therapy.

Clinical Hypothesis

I. Identifying information: Patient's name, age, schedule of appointments, communication disorder.

II. Background information: Brief accounts of patient's background and history including pertinent information about family, developmental, medical, educational, psychological, occupational, and treatment histories. Note current interests, activities, and talents.

III. Recent diagnostic results: Brief statement of patient's most recent evaluation and test results.

IV. Statement of the problem: Brief statement of the particular clinical problem to be treated.

V. Treatment goals: Statement of behaviors patient is expected to achieve.

VI. Rationale for treatment goals: Reasons for choosing these goals (why the goals are appropriate for this patient).

VII. Methodology: List of procedures and materials to use to achieve the patient's treatment goals.

VIII. Rationale for methodology: Reason for choosing these procedures and materials.

IX. Bibliography: References from the literature to support the above hypothesis.

   The only way to confirm a hypothesis is to eliminate alternative hypotheses. Simply making and verifying predictions are not the best ways to confirm a hypothesis. Make predictions with alternate hypotheses in mind, so as to eliminate as many of these hypotheses as possible. The hypothesis gains strength by defeating logical and reasonable alternatives, much like a champion athlete becomes an "all-time great" by defeating exceptionally strong challenges by rivals.

Empirical confirmation requires that the scientist or clinician always regard explanatory statements as tentative, seek new ways to test them against observations and other explanations, and never accept them as final truths.

The Scientific Method versus "Common Sense"

This section uses Anderson's (1971) model, with changes to make it relevant to communication sciences and disorders. By *common sense* we mean patterns of thoughts that are both widespread and unscientific. This is also referred to as *fallacious reasoning* or what *not* to do according to the scientific method.

Psychological Verification

A descriptive statement is considered to be true if it is authoritative, comforting, or familiar. Empirical verification requires that we observe, but the principle of psychological verification tells us not to observe. The corollaries suggest ways to avoid observation. In empirical observation we try to find consistencies among explanatory statements and between explanatory and descriptive statements, but in psychological verification we are instructed not to think logically (better yet, not to think at all) about relationships among statements.

The essential point is to avoid the test of observation, because it is difficult, cumbersome, and time consuming to apply. We may be forced to discard some fine thoughts merely because they are not supported by facts. Common-sense reasoning, therefore, is to avoid any test that might not support the desired outcome.

The Test of Authority

Focus on the authority figure, rather than statements or evidence. In this way, we can accept each authoritative statement without being concerned about truth or falsity. We can decide in advance to accept or reject future statements based on our evaluation of the authority figure. Evaluation criteria might include prestige, power, wealth, and personal confidence. If the authority is a group, the criterion might be the size of the group. For example, you should believe what you just read, because the authors are experts in their fields.

The Test of Comfort

This is also known as *wishful thinking*, in that we accept pleasant statements and reject those that are unpleasant. For example, global warming might be a good thing, because it reduces the harshness of winters. Feelings of hate, anger, or fear are justified as the responses of righteous people to wrongdoing by others. As an example, children with Down syndrome may be thought to be docile and sweet, whereas children with autism may be considered distant and difficult.

The Test of Familiarity

We accept familiar statements and reject those that are unfamiliar. Advertisements are repeated so often that they must contain at least a germ of truth. People with brain damage are "vegetables" and those who are deaf are also "dumb," according to the test of familiarity.

Anderson (1971) suggested the following principles as ways of avoiding the test of observations, in other words, avoiding the scientific method.

Verbal Definition

If terms in a descriptive statement are undefined or defined in strictly verbal terms, then they avoid testability.

Use Vague Terms

Terms that are sufficiently vague in their reference to observations will not be useful in determining truth or falsity of statements in which they are used. For example, it is impossible to insult elderly individuals with Alzheimer disease, because they don't care if you do.

Use Verbal Definitions

When required to define terms, substitute one set of operationally vague terms for another. Explain that the child who does not attend to a task must lack focus.

Use Circular Statements

For example, stuttering is everything you do to stop stuttering. An individual who continues to stutter didn't stop trying to stop stuttering.

Attach a "Nonobservability" Clause

The phenomenon will not appear if it is being looked at. For example, write in your diagnostic report that the only time the child hears normally is when it is absolutely quiet.

Uncontrolled Observation

When the test of observation must be applied, it can be made more flexible by inferring causality from natural co-occurrences or naturally occurring correlations. The definition of *post hoc ergo propter hoc* reasoning (after this therefore because of this) is: If B follows A, then A is the cause of B. The child with hyperfunctional voice disorder became hoarse after attending a baseball game, so the parents are counseled to discontinue taking the child to any more games.

Overgeneralization

Once you have arrived at a conclusion, generalize it as broadly as possible. Don't burden your conclusions with restrictions and qualifications. If you state the conclusion simply enough, then there will be no need for further observations.

Generalize to Unexamined Values of Independent Variables

For example, ASHA membership is growing at an astounding rate. The number of ASHA members quadrupled from 1980 to 2000. If the number keeps quadrupling every 20 years, there should be nearly a half million ASHA members by 2020 and more ASHA members than people in about 150 years.

Generalize to Unexamined Values of Sampled Variables

This is a method for extending conclusions. If you prepare an individualized educational plan (IEP) for a child with a language disorder, the same IEP should be useful for all other children with language disorders (see, for example, the "gray book" for preparing an IEP).

Generalize to Unexamined Values of Controlled Variables

This is reasoning by analogy. For example, M&Ms have been used as effective reinforcers in behavior modification studies with children in the autistic spectrum. Extend this conclusion to use chocolate in dysphagia management treatments.

Generalize to Different Operational Definitions of Variables

Many bilingual Spanish-English tests have been standardized using Spanish-speaking children living in Mexico. If you are testing a child who learned Spanish in any of the other 21 countries where Spanish is spoken, you should not be concerned about this.

Psychological Confirmation

Once you accept an explanatory statement, you never need to reject it. You can deal with inconsistencies found in other statements by discarding or altering the competing statements or by ignoring or modifying the relationships between them. Because your awareness of inconsistency is the result of thinking, not of observation, then the solution is either:

1. do not think or
2. if you must, think very carefully.

Do Not Think

Ignore One of the Ideas or the Relationship between Them. Repression is a well-known and time-tested way of dealing with conflicting ideas. If deaf children are convinced by their elders that cochlear implants represent a betrayal of their Deaf community, then they will be less likely to think about the consequences of being able to hear.

Logic-Tight Compartmentalization. Keep ideas from coming into contact, so you can think about them both. For example, you are charitable on the Sabbath, and find it reasonable to charge exorbitant fees during the week.

Think Carefully (If You Must Think)

Produce an Appearance of Compatibility. Modify one of the ideas or the relationship between them. Psychologists call this thinking *rationalization*; another term is *whitewash thinking*. There are two ways to modify one of two conflicting ideas to make it appear compatible with the other:

- Differentiating. Split the idea into two. If the caregiver's report does not correspond with your findings on a diagnostic test, then indicate that the caregiver is not a reliable informant.
- Bolstering. Change your attitude toward one idea so that it seems more congruent with the other. In "sour grapes" thinking, we emphasize undesirable aspects of the issue. If a client is hard to test, say he couldn't be conditioned. In "sweet lemon" thinking, we emphasize the desirable aspects. If you use facilitated communication, you have a heightened interest in articles that extol its virtues.

The Scientific Method and Pseudoscience

Finn et al. (2005) provide warning signs that alert a consumer or student that a claim may only appear to be scientific. The more such signs are in evidence, the greater the likelihood that the assertion, belief, or treatment approach is pseudoscientific. The article highlights 10 criteria that differentiate between science and pseudoscience. We describe below the six that refer to the quality of evidence used to support a treatment claim.

Untestable

Finn et al. (2005) ask if the treatment is not able to be tested or falsified. There are legitimate academic pursuits, such as theoretical linguistics, where models are never exposed to real-world tests. For example, assume the model called TPWSGWTAU (or *the place where sentences go when they are understood*). There is no intent to subject this model to empirical observation; indeed, any encounter it might have with data is unlikely to prove fatal. Rather, the model serves as a stimulus for empirical sciences to examine it further. Neurologists may study the brain structure of TPWSGWTAU; psychologists may consider processes leading to TPWSGWTAU.

Pseudoscience is exposed when there are claims of a treatment's benefits, but the claim is not testable or capable of being disproved. For example, all three judges found that efficacy of facilitated communication, a treatment sometimes used for autism, is not testable (Finn et al., 2005). Remember that these assertions or hypotheses may never be proven, because the treatments are applied to a sample rather than to the entire population. Theories may be strengthened if the results of empirical testing support the hypothetical construct, and they may be falsified or disproved if the treatment does not work as claimed. Other pseudoscientific claims are testable in principle, but are never tested in practice. Empirical tests that refute the claims are ignored or explained away with such generalities as, "No treatment works on everyone and everything."

Unchanged

Finn et al. (2005) ask if the treatment approach remains unchanged even if there is contradictory evidence. It is possible for a good treatment to have mistakes, misconceptions, or inaccuracies. For example, Melodic Intonation Therapy (MIT) is a well-known means of treating moderate nonfluent aphasia, based on the premise that the musical abilities of the undamaged right cerebral hemisphere can facilitate word retrieval after a stroke in the left hemisphere of the brain. However, the authors (Albert, Sparks, & Helm, 1973) erred in the protocol, which required their patients to shift from intoned forms of utterances to normal speech prosody. They recognized their error and instituted a transitional stage, called *sprechgesang* (speech-song), which bridged the gap between speaking and singing, resulting in an effective treatment.

Because pseudoscientific claims are not typically exposed to empirical testing, the errors are seldom self-corrected. The treatment of stuttering offers many examples of this type of pseudoscience. Relating the problem of stuttering to the structure of the individual's tongue is at least as old as Aristotle, and the claim found its avatar in the 1800s in Diefenbach, who performed partial glossectomies to "cure" stuttering. Removing the tongue would remove the stuttering. (We suppose it is fortunate that the same claim was not made for headaches.)

Confirming Evidence

Finn et al. (2005) ask if the rationale for the treatment approach was based only on confirming evidence, so that disconfirming evidence was ignored or minimized. Even a pseudoscientific treatment may garner some corroborating or confirming evidence. However, there are different levels of evidence. Positive results from a single therapy session with an individual client may be meaningful, but lack the force of results from randomized, double-blinded, placebo-controlled clinical trials replicated by independent investigators. It is a human frailty that we tend to assign greater credibility to evidence that confirms rather than disconfirms our beliefs. Pseudoscience is not the practice of only ignoring disconfirming evidence; rather than being receptive, even if evidence is disconfirming, pseudoscientists explain away the differences, and save the original idea by adding some ad hoc hypotheses that incorporate the new evidence.

The tendency to overemphasize confirming evidence is most apparent in studies where the researchers have a fiduciary interest in the outcome. That is, there is a monetary reward for confirming one's findings and a penalty for disconfirming them. Many scientific journals (ASHA's publications among them) require a disclosure statement from prospective contributors regarding a possible conflict of interest. It is important for consumers to know if they are reading reports of independent research versus research and development undertaken to bring a product to market.

Anecdotal Evidence

Finn et al. (2005) ask if the evidence supporting the treatment relies on personal experience and anecdotal accounts. Case study research is designed to examine in depth specific individuals or situations in order to illustrate important principles that might be overlooked in examining group data. For example, the relatively new syndrome of primary progressive aphasia was identified after a case study in Canada was followed by a decade of similar reports of cases around the world. Useful as they are, scientists recognize that case studies provide a weak foundation for making valid inferences about treatment. Proper examination of treatment efficacy, or evidence for clinical practice, requires experimental controls, which are not found in case studies.

Pseudoscience uses case studies, testimonials, and personal experiences as its bread and butter. The claim of repressed and recovered memories, popular a generation ago, resulted in well-meaning individuals testifying in court about events from decades earlier that they just recovered in memory. These testimonials threatened to result in the incarceration of innocent people, until the claims of repressed and recovered memories fell out of fashion. There are many threats to the validity (generalizability of the data) of an experiment, including practice effects and the placebo effect. We need to eliminate alternative explanations that might account for the treatment effects. The fewer the alternative explanations, the greater the internal validity of the experiment.

Inadequate Evidence

Finn et al. (2005) ask if treatment claims are not commensurate with the level of evidence required to support those claims. There is an old saying that extraordinary claims require extraordinary evidence. The purpose of research is no more or less than a search for a piece of truth. Note that the word *truth* includes a lowercase *t*. Outcome research follows phases, which address different questions using different methods. Eventually, it is possible that the pieces of lowercase *t* truths that are revealed are collected into a capital-*T* Truth.

Pseudoscience often jumps right into the upper case. Asserting a fundamental right to the Truth, pseudoscientists turn the process of discovery on its head, claiming that it is the responsibility of their critics to prove them wrong. The argument from this position of ignorance that a claim must be correct represents the kind of fallacious reasoning that is elaborated on in The Scientific Method versus "Common Sense," above.

Avoiding Peer Review

Finn et al. (2005) ask if treatment gains are unsupported by evidence that has been evaluated critically. The gold standard that evidence has undergone critical evaluation is publication in a peer-reviewed journal. The ASHA journals, including *Journal of Speech, Language, and Hearing Research*; *American Journal of Speech-Language Pathology*; *American Journal of Audiology*; and *Language, Speech, and Hearing Services in Schools*, are all peer-reviewed publications. Authors submit unsolicited articles to the editor of the journal, who forwards the material to an associate editor with expertise in the area of study. The associate editor requests three experts in the field (selected from volunteers who have previously been appointed to a review panel) to write a detailed critique of the paper. Recommendations for or against publication are generally in the four categories of accept, accept with minor revisions, accept with major revisions, and reject. The journal editor makes the final determination, and forwards the critical evaluations to the authors.

The peer-review process may be subverted by reviewers who wish to promote a particular agenda, style, or method of research. Even when the peer review is putatively blind, with reviewers and authors remaining anonymous, it is not uncommon for reviewers to recognize the work of scholars from laboratories that may be competing with the reviewers' for funding and recognition. Similarly, authors whose work has been rejected from journals with the most rigorous review process can often find a home for their work, even if it is in an on-line journal where authors are responsible for submitting their own external peer reviews (presumably from sympathetic friends).

Papers that are self-published, either in hard copy or on the Internet, have not undergone peer review. Pseudoscientific approaches to treatment may be promoted directly to the public, often very effectively, through advertisements or stories that emphasize emotional rather than intellectual content. The scientific process of peer review should include challenges to claims that may be one-sided or biased, whereas the pseudoscientific approach is less likely to do so.

Evaluation of Student's Evidence-Based Writing in Speech-Language Pathology

The following is edited from an actual report. Correct the examples of incorrect usage. Each item is followed by a number in parentheses. Answers follow.

Clinical hypothesis. A phonological approach will improve production of postvocalic /t/ and /p/ more than a traditional approach in a preschool male.

Client profile. Z.Z. is a three year, four month old (1) male who presents with a speech delay. Observations indicate that he omits the final /p/ and /t/ sounds in words. His mother expressed concern that he did not finish the endings of his words. His mother also added that his immediate family understands him, but other adults often display difficulty understanding his speech.

Pre-treatment baseline data. The following data was (2) collected prior to initiation of his treatment program: The client was producing the final /t/ sound in words with 40% accuracy. The client was producing the final /p/ sound in words with 50 % accuracy. (3)

Treatment technique. The clinician used an alternating treatment approach for a single subject. (4) The two treatments used during therapy included a phonological approach and a traditional approach. The clinician used minimal pairs during phonological therapy to emphasize the consonants at the end of words. The client refused to participate in this task. Whether due to lack of interest, (5) or the unability (6) to comprehend this goal, this approach was discarded. (7) The remaining therapy sessions focused on the traditional approach. The techniques used during traditional articulation therapy included modeling, direct imitation, and motor exercises. These techniques, as well as visual prompts, elicited the final /t/ and /p/ sounds at the word, phrase, and sentence levels.

Treatment efficacy evidence. Klein (1996) observed that a study indicated that children who received traditional therapy did not perform as well as children who received phonological therapy. The children in the phonological group were all released from therapy, whereas only two of the children (8) in the traditional therapy group reached age-appropriate speech.

Data following 10 weeks of treatment. The client produced the final /p/ in words with 90% accuracy and the final /t/ in words with 85% accuracy. (9)

Conclusion. Results suggest that traditional therapy is improving Z.Z.'s intelligibility by emphasizing the final /T/ and /P/ (10) in words, with carryover observed at the phrase and sentence levels.

Reference

Klein, E. S. (1996). Phonological/traditional approaches to articulation therapy: A retrospective group comparison. *Language, Speech, and Hearing Services in Schools, 27,* 314–323.

ANSWERS

1. Use numerals and hyphens as follows: "Z.Z. is a 3-year, 4-month-old male . . . "

2. *Data* is a plural word (singular is *datum*). Accordingly, "The following data *were* collected."

3. The statement of *50% accuracy* is inadequate without also including the number of trials. The reader does not know if there were 5 correct responses out of 10 or 50 out of 100.

4. The word *subject* should be changed to *client* if, as in the present case, the context is therapy, or changed to *participant* if the context is an experiment.

5. It would be better to indicate, in behavioral terms, how the client showed lack of interest.

6. The word *inability* was misspelled.

7. The sentence has poor syntax. Without specifying the client or the clinician as the subject of the sentence, *the approach*, which should be the object of the sentence, becomes the subject. This does not make sense.

8. It is meaningless to report that two children reached criterion in the study cited without indicating the total number in the sample: 2 out of 2 is very different from 2 out of 10.

9. As in 3, the report of percent correct should also include number of trials. In addition, it would be helpful to indicate the number of treatment sessions where the criterion applied. Instead of merely reporting 85% accuracy, it would be much more meaningful to indicate 85% accuracy in 20 trials over three consecutive therapy sessions, or 17/20 correct for three consecutive sessions.

10. Phonemes are always written in the lower case, as in /t/ and /p/, not /T/ and /P/.

References

Albert, M., Sparks, R., & Helm, N. (1973). Melodic intonation therapy for aphasia. *Archives of Neurology, 29*, 130–131.

American Speech-Language-Hearing Association. (2005). Evidence-based practice in communication disorders [Position statement]. Available at http://www.asha.org/docs/html/PS2005-00221.html

Anderson, B. F. (1971). *The psychology experiment.* Belmont, CA: Brooks/Cole.

Finn, P., Bothe, A. K., & Bramlett, R. E. (2005). Science and pseudoscience in communication disorders: Criteria and applications. *American Journal of Speech-Language Pathology, 14*, 172–186.

Santo Pietro, M. J., & Goldfarb, R. (1995). *Techniques for aphasia rehabilitation generating effective treatment (TARGET).* Vero Beach, FL: The Speech Bin.

Schuell, H., Jenkins, J., & Jimenez-Pabon, E. (1964). *Aphasia in adults: Diagnosis, prognosis, and treatment.* New York: Hoeber Medical Division, Harper.

EXERCISES

1. Which is the best source of evidence, and why?
   a. Information found on http://www.asha.org
   b. Information from your professor in a graduate course
   c. Information from the *Journal of Speech, Language, and Hearing Research*
   d. Information from a presentation at a state SLP/A convention
   e. Information from you own clinical experience

2. The fallacy of *post hoc ergo propter hoc* is represented in which of the statements?
   a. Aphasia is caused by a stroke.
   b. Conductive hearing loss is caused by cleft palate.
   c. Loss of hair cells in the cochlea causes sensorineural hearing loss.
   d. There is no general agreement about what causes stuttering.
   e. If B follows A, then A follows B.

3. Explain what is wrong with this definition: Stuttering is everything you do to stop stuttering.

4. Explain what is wrong with this statement: If you see a young child with conductive hearing loss, you will also see evidence of middle ear infection.

ANSWERS

1. The best source of evidence would come from a peer-reviewed journal, so the correct answer is *c*. Professional Web sites, even our own (choice *a*) and convention presentations (choice *d*) are more likely to include up-to-the-minute information. What is most current is often not sufficiently vetted, so information from these sources should be considered work in progress. Although one's professor (choice *b*) is ethically obliged to tell the truth and stay current with professional literature, the student needs to be aware that some information might be based on psychological verification, and not always empirical verification. Because clinical experience involves a small population of individuals with a particular disorder, generalizability is limited.

2. The *post hoc* fallacy is represented in *b*. Individuals with cleft palate frequently have conductive hearing loss, but the cleft does not cause it. There is general agreement that a stroke causes aphasia (choice *a*), just as there is no single unifying explanation for stuttering (choice *d*). There is a causal relation between loss of cochlear hair cells and sensorineural loss of hearing (choice *c*). *Post hoc ergo propter hoc* is expressed as follows: If B follows A, then A is the cause of B.

3. The problem has to do with verbal (as opposed to operational) definition. You should not use the term to be defined (in this case, *stuttering*) in the definition.

4. The problem is overgeneralization. Many children with conductive hearing loss do not have middle ear infection, and many children with middle ear infection do not have conductive hearing loss.

CHAPTER 3

Ethics of Professional Writing

In Chapter 4 on writing using Internet resources, we identify several areas of ethical concern in research. The focus of the present chapter is on ethical considerations in professional and clinical writing.

By *ethics* we mean moral decision making. A too-common example of an ethical lapse is the discussion of patients by medical personnel that we overhear when riding in the hospital elevator. Imagine the pain of a visitor who hears an intern casually indicate to a colleague that the visitor's relative "isn't going to make it."

We begin this chapter with an annotated Code of Ethics, continue with a discussion of relevant legal guidelines regarding ethical practice, and conclude with a sample form for compliance with ethical standards.

The ASHA Code of Ethics

The American Speech-Language-Hearing Association (ASHA) began a nearly 2½-year process of revising its *Code of Ethics* in August 2000, focusing on ethics in research and professional practice. The revised *Code of Ethics* took effect on January 1, 2003 (reprinted by permission from ASHA). The Preamble begins as follows:

> The preservation of the highest standards of integrity and ethical principles is vital to the responsible discharge of obligations by speech-language pathologists, audiologists, and speech,

language, and hearing scientists. This Code of Ethics sets forth
the fundamental principles and rules considered essential to
this purpose.

In annotating parts of the *Code of Ethics*, the authors are attempting to highlight only those portions that refer to clinical and professional practice, and to omit those portions that refer to research or
treatment of animals. We have used elisions (three periods separated
by spaces) to indicate portions omitted, and brackets to add a word
for grammatical purposes when elisions affected sentence structure.
The editorial opinions of the authors will be preceded by *Comment.*

Principle of Ethics I

Individuals shall honor their responsibility to hold paramount
the welfare of persons they serve professionally.

Comment: The revisions in Principle of Ethics I add humane treatment of animals to the section on welfare of research participants
and also address issues of nondiscrimination, informed consent,
confidentiality, and security of research data.

Rules of Ethics

A. Individuals shall provide all services competently.

Comment: ASHA members who hold the Certificate of Clinical
Competence (CCC) have, by virtue of completing an advanced
degree from an accredited college or university, passing the
national examination in speech-language pathology or audiology,
and completing the supervised Clinical Fellowship, demonstrated the ability to provide competent services. Should ASHA
members with the CCC be considered competent in all areas
of clinical practice? Many newly licensed and certified speech-
language pathologists have never earned practicum hours with
clients who have fluency or voice disorders; are they equipped
to treat stuttering or spasmodic dysphonia? Few students in
audiology are ever provided with clinical training in interoper-
ative monitoring; are they qualified to perform and interpret
auditory evoked measures during surgical procedures?

B. Individuals shall use every resource, including referral when appropriate, to ensure that high-quality service is provided.

Comment: Rule B answers the comment raised in A, and requires that individuals without proper education, training, or experience in a particular area of communication disorders refer clients with such disorders to a practitioner with proper education, training, and experience. Offering credentials in specialization areas will facilitate appropriate referrals.

C. Individuals shall not discriminate in the delivery of professional services . . . on the basis of race or ethnicity, gender, age, religion, national origin, sexual orientation, or disability.

Comment: None.

D. Individuals shall not misrepresent the credentials of assistants, technicians, or support personnel and shall inform those they serve professionally of the name and professional credentials of persons providing services.

Comment: Student clinicians should sign their names above the title "Clinical Intern," or a similar designation approved by the institution, on all diagnostic evaluations, daily log notes, progress reports, and clinical summaries. The clinical supervisor who holds full credentials should also sign these documents.

E. Individuals who hold the Certificates of Clinical Competence shall not delegate tasks that require the unique skills, knowledge, and judgment that are within the scope of their profession to assistants, technicians, support personnel, students, or any nonprofessionals over whom they have supervisory responsibility. An individual may delegate support services to assistants, technicians, support personnel, students, or any other persons only if those services are adequately supervised by an individual who holds the appropriate Certificate of Clinical Competence.

Comment: According to Council of Academic Accreditation (CAA) standards, student clinicians are required to be directly supervised by an individual holding the CCC for 25% of therapy time and 50% of diagnostic time. By signing a student's hourly log and affixing the ASHA account number, the supervisor guarantees that these requirements have been met or exceeded.

F. Individuals shall fully inform the persons they serve of the nature and possible effects of services rendered and products dispensed. . .

Comment: An audiologist must provide effective counseling to patients on expectations with amplification. Hearing aids function as sound amplifiers that indiscriminately enhance sound signals, including undesirable background noise. Counseling in addition to a listening adjustment period for users is therefore necessary for a successful hearing aid fitting.

G. Individuals shall evaluate the effectiveness of services rendered and of products dispensed and shall provide services or dispense products only when benefit can reasonably be expected.

Comment: Understanding the differences between science and pseudoscience in communication disorders will facilitate critical evaluation of controversial practices and products, as Finn, Bothe, and Bramlett (2005) do with facilitated communication and Fast ForWord, as well as with the SpeechEasy device.

H. Individuals shall not guarantee the results of any treatment or procedure, directly or by implication; however, they may make a reasonable statement of prognosis.

Comment: In fitting a hearing aid, an audiologist may anticipate that the patient's amplified hearing may approach typical levels, but may not state that the device will restore normal hearing.

I. Individuals shall not provide clinical services solely by correspondence.

Comment: None.

J. Individuals may practice by telecommunication (for example, telehealth/e-health), where not prohibited by law.

Comment: Although individual practitioners typically hold the CCC, they are required in most cases to be licensed by the state in which they practice. State laws supersede rules of ethics in regard to Rule J.

K. Individuals shall adequately maintain and appropriately secure records of professional services rendered. . . and products dispensed and shall allow access to these records only when authorized or when required by law.

Comment: See the section on the Health Insurance Portability and Accountability Act of 1996 (HIPAA) for elaboration.

L. Individuals shall not reveal, without authorization, any professional or personal information about identified persons served professionally . . . unless required by law to do so, or unless doing so is necessary to protect the welfare of the person or of the community or otherwise required by law.

Comment: Individually identifiable health information is protected by HIPAA.

M. Individuals shall not charge for services not rendered, nor shall they misrepresent services rendered [or] products dispensed . . .

Comment: None.

N. Individuals shall use persons . . . as subjects of teaching demonstrations only with their informed consent.

Comment: Student clinicians should obtain release forms for video- and audio-taping before beginning therapy. These forms should indicate that tapes and other information will be used for teaching purposes only.

O. Individuals whose professional services are adversely affected by substance abuse or other health-related conditions shall seek professional assistance and, where appropriate, withdraw from the affected areas of practice.

Comment: Student clinicians with the above conditions should notify the clinical supervisor and the clinic director. In some cases, affected student clinicians might also contact the university office of mental health or disability services. When the health-related condition is a pregnancy, the student clinician should advise the persons in charge of internship and externship placements if delivery is expected midsemester.

Principle of Ethics II

Individuals shall honor their responsibility to achieve and maintain the highest level of professional competence.

Comment: Principle of Ethics II refers to professional competency. The philosophy articulated by ASHA parallels that of hospitals, where physicians may have general, specialized, or research privileges (Goldfarb, 1989). Research and specialized privileges include all general privileges and responsibilities. Specialized privileges, such as evaluating a client's suitability for a cochlear implant or an alternative-augmentative communication device, are earned through additional credentialing, coursework, or continuing education.

Rules of Ethics

A. Individuals shall engage in the provision of clinical services only when they hold the appropriate Certificate of Clinical Competence or when they are in the certification process and are supervised by an individual who holds the appropriate Certificate of Clinical Competence.

Comment: The United States Bureau of Labor Statistics has listed the professions of speech-language pathology and audiology among the leading growth professions for the coming decade (and has done so for many years). The shortage of fully credentialed practitioners has led some employers, particularly school districts, to appeal for and be granted exemption from the *highest quality provider* requirement of the state. Nevertheless, ASHA is exercising moral decision making by stipulating the CCC as a minimum requirement for best practice.

B. Individuals shall engage in only those aspects of the professions that are within the scope of their competence, considering their level of education, training, and experience.

Comment: This rule is similar to, and was addressed in, comments to Rules IA and IB.

C. Individuals shall continue their professional development throughout their careers.

Comment: The professions of speech-language pathology and audiology require lifelong learning for maintaining and developing new knowledge and skills. Although ASHA and most states require completion of 30 hours of continuing education every 3 years, many ASHA members, including the present authors, have earned ASHA's Award for Continuing Education (ACE), which requires completion of 70 hours of continuing education in 3 years.

D. Individuals shall delegate the provision of clinical services only to: (1) persons who hold the appropriate Certificate of Clinical Competence; (2) persons in the education or certification process who are appropriately supervised by an individual who holds the appropriate Certificate of Clinical Competence; or (3) assistants, technicians, or support personnel who are adequately supervised by an individual who holds the appropriate Certificate of Clinical Competence.

Comment: Employees in exempt settings (see IIA above) are, we submit, ethically bound to abide by Rule IID, even if they are not legally bound to do so. Log notes, reports, and letters written by individuals without the CCC should indicate the status of the provider, such as "student intern," and be countersigned by the CCC-level supervisor.

E. Individuals shall not require or permit their professional staff to provide services . . . that exceed the staff member's competence, level of education, training, and experience.

Comment: One of the more sensitive issues of ethics is coercion. The possibility of staff members who are unsure of their job security being tyrannized by a coercive director is, of course, of ethical concern. Of equal concern is the staff member who considers the individual in charge to be a mentor. Whenever there is a power differential, the individual in the position of power must be especially sensitive to the possibility of perhaps unintended coercion. See Schmidt, Galletta, and Obler (2006) for more information on coercion and power differentials.

F. Individuals shall ensure that all equipment used in the provision of services . . . is in proper working order and is properly calibrated.

Comment: The effectiveness of clinical services is dependent upon on the accurate performance of any equipment used to perform them. Clinicians who rely on the use of equipment in service delivery must systematically assess the equipment function according to manufacturer specifications, and at minimum, ASHA guidelines. In audiology, where there is a heavy reliance on equipment for most services, biologic (listening), quarterly, and annual calibrations are routinely performed in order to ascertain proper equipment function.

Principle of Ethics III

Individuals shall honor their responsibility to the public by promoting public understanding of the professions, by supporting the development of services designed to fulfill the unmet needs of the public, and by providing accurate information in all communications involving any aspect of the professions . . .

Comment: Revisions in Principle of Ethics III relate to accurate and honest information about an individual's contributions to scholarly and research activities.

Rules of Ethics

A. Individuals shall not misrepresent their credentials, competence, education, training, experience, or scholarly or research contributions.

Comment: We knew of an individual who described himself as a neuroaudiologist, a title which does not exist. ASHA will need to be clear about which new titles will be permissible with specialized credentialing (e.g., Will "board-certified aphasiologist" be acceptable?).

B. Individuals shall not participate in professional activities that constitute a conflict of interest.

Comment: As with coercion, conflict of interest is a subtle and thorny issue. When the first author directed a PhD program, the faculty engaged in some stimulating discussions. In one case, we resolved that it would be a conflict of interest for a doctoral student to engage in dissertation research at a paid employment site, unless the employment was a research fellowship. In another case, we permitted a student who had not yet earned CCC to undertake a clinical externship with a supervisor who did not have a PhD. We were concerned that the supervisor might be considering pursuing a doctoral degree at our program, and that placing one of our students in an externship might be coercive. It also might be a conflict of interest if the individual decided to apply for admission to the doctoral program while serving as a supervisor.

C. Individuals shall refer those served professionally solely on the basis of the interest of those being referred and not on any personal financial interest.

Comment: It is accepted practice in the legal profession to pay a substantial referral fee when, for example, an attorney specializing in accidental injuries assigns one third of the contingency fee to the referring attorney in general practice. Such practice is ethically proscribed in the professions of speech-language pathology and audiology.

D. Individuals shall not misrepresent diagnostic information, research, services rendered, or products dispensed; neither shall they engage in any scheme to defraud in connection with obtaining payment or reimbursement for such services or products.

Comment: (See Chapter 7 for information about writing the diagnostic report.) Digital signal processing is considered a technological advancement over analog hearing aid circuits. In the 1990s when digital hearing aid processing became clinically available, there was a considerable price differentiation between the existing (analog) and very expensive new technology. Clinical studies at that time, however, did not support significantly better performance outcomes for patients fitted with digital as compared to analog hearing aids. It would therefore have been unethical to recommend a digital device to a client on the basis that it is "better" in terms of hearing improvement over a comparable analog device.

E. Individuals' statements to the public shall provide accurate information about the nature and management of communication disorders, about the professions, [and] about professional services . . .

Comment: Any written or oral statements made by student clinicians, in the form of a press release, advertisement, or interview, should be vetted by the clinic director, as well as approved through the chain of command, which might include the program director, department chair, divisional dean, and university offices of information services or institutional advancement. This should take place even if the written or oral statement refers to an externship facility.

F. Individuals' statements to the public—advertising, announcing, and marketing their professional services, . . . and promoting products—shall adhere to prevailing professional standards and shall not contain misrepresentation.

Comment: Approvals through the chain of command indicated for Rule IIIE apply to IIIF as well.

Principle of Ethics IV

Individuals shall honor their responsibilities to the professions and their relationships with colleagues, students, and members of allied professions. Individuals shall uphold the dignity and autonomy of the professions, maintain harmonious interprofessional and extraprofessional relationships, and accept the professions' self-imposed standards.

Comment: The rule of law prevails, but rules of ethics may hold a higher standard. The ethical rules that follow, presented without comment, include proscriptions previously discussed, which include deceit, coercion, conflict of interest, and abuse of power.

Rules of Ethics

A. Individuals shall prohibit anyone under their supervision from engaging in any practice that violates the Code of Ethics.

B. Individuals shall not engage in dishonesty, fraud, deceit, misrepresentation, sexual harassment, or any other form of conduct that adversely reflects on the professions or on the individual's fitness to serve persons professionally.

C. Individuals shall not engage in sexual activities with clients or students over whom they exercise professional authority.

D. Individuals shall assign credit only to those who have contributed to a publication, presentation, or product. Credit shall be assigned in proportion to the contribution and only with the contributor's consent.

E. Individuals shall reference the source when using other person's ideas, research, presentations, or products in written, oral, or any other media presentation or summary.

F. Individuals' statements to colleagues about professional services, research results, and products shall adhere to prevailing professional standards and shall contain no misrepresentations.

G. Individuals shall not provide professional services without exercising independent professional judgment, regardless of referral source or prescription.

H. Individuals shall not discriminate in their relationships with colleagues, students, and members of allied professions on the basis of race or ethnicity, gender, age, religion, national origin, sexual orientation, or disability.

I. Individuals who have reason to believe that the Code of Ethics has been violated shall inform the Board of Ethics.

J. Individuals shall comply fully with the policies of the Board of Ethics in its consideration and adjudication of complaints of violations of the Code of Ethics.

Final Comment: The *ASHA Leader* will occasionally report members who have violated one or more rules in the *Code of Ethics*. The principles and rules violated will be cited, as well as the punishment for the violation.

Health Insurance Portability and Accountability Act of 1996 (HIPAA)

Consider the following scenario: Your mother (or father, sibling, or spouse) has just come out of surgery. You call the hospital for an update and are told that you are not authorized to receive any information about the patient. You should:

1. scream indignantly, "But it's my mother (father, sibling, spouse)!"
2. threaten to sue,
3. sob hysterically, or
4. be grateful that your loved one's medical confidentiality is being protected.

HIPAA was established by the 104th Congress on August 21, 1996, as Public Law 104-191, which amended the Internal Revenue Code of 1986. The purpose of the new law was to combat waste, fraud, and abuse in health care delivery. The function of HIPAA was to establish standards and requirements for electronic transmission of health information and to encourage the development of a health information system.

Many aspects of HIPAA are relevant to students and practitioners in communication sciences and disorders. The term *health information* refers to oral or recorded forms, created by a health care provider (including a speech-language pathologist or audiologist), school, or university, which address the physical or mental health of an individual in the present, past, or future.

Confidentiality protection under HIPAA refers to individually identifiable health information. Any demographic or other physical or mental health information that can reasonably be believed to identify a person is included. The 16-page document addresses security standards and safeguards, such as keeping confidential records in locked file cabinets in locked rooms away from waiting areas.

There are monetary and incarceration penalties for failure to comply with HIPAA requirements and standards. In addition, the site visit team from ASHA's Council on Academic Accreditation will determine if confidentiality protections are enforced by a college or university speech and hearing center before awarding accreditation to that program. Finally, some third-party payers will refuse payment to a speech and hearing center that does not provide adequate documentation and protection of health information.

The Institutional Review Board

There is a laudable trend in graduate and even some undergraduate programs in communication sciences and disorders (CSD) to require students to present documentation of their evidence-based (research-based) clinical practice (see Chapter 2). Some programs set aside an evening for student presentations as a poster session, with invitations sent throughout the university and even the neighboring community. Students stay next to their posters and answer questions, as visitors circulate among the many impressive presentations. This project serves many functions:

1. It serves to reinforce the clinician-researcher connection.
2. It advertises the excellent work of the speech and hearing center.
3. It highlights the achievements of CSD students to members of the department, school, and university.

The project also raises some ethical questions:

1. How will confidentiality of participants be ensured?
2. How have ethical standards of treatment for human participants been assured?
   a. Safety and appropriateness of research methodology
   b. Informed consent
3. How has potential for coercion in the supervisor-student or mentor-student relationship been avoided?

Some of the ethical questions have already been addressed in this chapter. For example, HIPAA is concerned with issues of confidentiality, and the ASHA Code of Ethics sets limits on the types of interactions, even friendships, permitted in supervisor-student and mentor-student relationships. Another level of ethical protection is provided by the Institutional Review Board (IRB). Clinicians and students engaging in clinical research that will be submitted for presentation at a poster session must write a proposal for approval by the IRB.

The Hammurabi code of "First, do no harm" is usually cited as the beginning of patient welfare concern (Schwartz, 2006). Compare this code to the "experiments" conducted by physicians in Nazi Germany, which led to the Nuremberg Code. At the end of World War II, the Nuremberg Military Tribunal established standards for research and conduct with human participants. These standards must also be applied in the clinical intervention conducted in our speech and hearing centers. They include:

1. Voluntary consent. The participant must also have the capacity to consent, the consent has to be given without direct or indirect coercion, and the participant must understand the risks and benefits of the treatment. The participant's age or degree of impairment may require an advocate to approve the treatment. For example, a participant

or advocate must understand that there may be discomfort (i.e., elicited dizziness) associated with portions of vestibular electronystagmography (ENG) testing, or that there may be a risk of aspiration associated with the treatment of dysphagia.
2. Risk-to-benefit ratio. The ratio must be favorable to the participant, with risks minimized, and the participant is permitted to withdraw from treatment at any time.

The Belmont Report

In 1979, the *Belmont Report* set out three core ethical principles for human participants in research. We have extended them to include participants in clinical intervention. The Belmont Report Historical Archive is available (subject to change) at http://www.hhs.gov/ohrp/belmontArchive.html and includes interviews with participants of the National Commission for the Protection of Human Subjects of Biomedical and Behavioral Research (1974–1978). There is also a 9-minute video, featuring participants of the commission.

1. Respect for persons. Individuals have the right to decide whether or not they wish to participate in treatment or research. These decisions should be based on full information and free from coercion.
2. Beneficence. The researcher or clinician has an obligation to minimize possible harm and to maximize potential benefits.
3. Justice. Benefits and risks of research and treatment should be fairly distributed across the population, as well as be fairly applied to individuals. For example, a drug currently in clinical trials (pagoclone, a GABA receptor modulator) may be effective in controlling stuttering. If efficacy is adequately demonstrated, the drug must be distributed according to the ethical principles identified in the *Belmont Report*.

National Institutes of Health (NIH) Training Course

Clinical writing may lead to professional and research writing. Any individual submitting a grant proposal to the National Institutes of Health (NIH; effective 2000) has been required to complete a computer-based training course on the protection of human research participants. The on-line course may be accessed by NIH employees (subject to change) at http://ohsr.od.nih.gov or, for individuals who are not employed by NIH (subject to change), at http://cme .cancer.gov/clinicaltrials/learning/humanparticipant-protections .asp. The course takes about 1 hour and permits the printing of a certificate of completion. It is an excellent overview of research ethics, and should be completed by anyone providing clinical intervention to human participants.

Conclusion

Before beginning any clinical research project involving human beings, the investigator (even if it is a student taking a clinical practicum course) must obtain approval from the Institutional Review Board. Forms are reasonably standard across institutions (see Chapter Appendix, sample IRB form, adapted from Adelphi University), and require a brief description of the project's purposes, methodology, and design; dates for initiation and completion of the project; number and characteristics of participants; method of recruitment; and any potential risks, stresses, or discomforts and the precautions taken to minimize them. Investigators must include an informed consent form and a representative sample of materials. There may also be a required debriefing form, as well as a sign-up sheet or advertisement.

References

American Speech-Language-Hearing Association. (2003). Code of ethics. *ASHA Supplement, 23,* 13–15.

Dillon, H. (2001). *Hearing aids.* New York: Thieme.

Finn, P., Bothe, A. K., & Bramlett, R. E. (2005). Science and pseudoscience in communication disorders: Criteria and applications. *American Journal of Speech-Language Pathology, 14,* 172–186.

Goldfarb, R. (1989). Organization of speech, language, and hearing programmes in United States hospitals. *The College of Speech Therapists Bulletin, 452,* 2–7.

Health Insurance Portability and Accountability Act (HIPAA) of 1996. Public Law 104–191, 104th Congress.

New York State Department of State Division of Licensing Services. Registration of Hearing Aid Dispensers 2001. General Business Law, Article 37-A.

Office for Protection from Research Risks, Protection of Human Subjects. National Commision for the Protection of Human Subjects of Biomedical and Behavioral Research. (1979). *The Belmont Report: Ethical principles and guidelines for the protections of human subjects of research* (GPO Office 887–890). Washington, DC: Government Printing Office.

Schmidt, B., Galleta, E., & Obler, L. K. (2006). Teaching research ethics in communi-cation disorders programs. In R. Goldfarb (Ed.), *Ethics: A case study from fluency* (pp. 63–82). San Diego, CA: Plural.

Schwartz, R. G. (2006). Would today's IRB approve the Tudor study? Ethical considerations in conducting research involving children with communication disorders. In R. Goldfarb (Ed.), *Ethics: A case study from fluency* (pp. 83–96). San Diego, CA: Plural.

Wilber, L. A. (2002). Calibration: Puretone, speech, and noise signals. In J. Katz (Ed.), *Handbook of clinical audiology* (pp. 50–70). Baltimore: Lippincott Williams &Wilkins.

EXERCISES

1. Correct the writing and the ethical errors in the following letter to a former professor:

   January 1, 2009

   Hey Dr. G,

   I'm going on a job interview next week and I need your help. If you could write me a letter of recommendation. The supervisor of speech wants to go for a doctorate at Adelphi, and you would certainly have some leverage as the program director, if you say she should hire me, she probably would, because she wants to make a favorable impression on you.

   Thanks.

   Sincerely,
   Will di Sappoint

2. Scandinavicon, a new manufacturer of digital hearing aids, is offering free trips to its flagship store in Copenhagen. United States-based audiologists who have active practices including prescribing hearing aids are invited to apply to participate in a weekend conference in Denmark on Scandinavicon aids, with all expenses paid. Should you apply? What should you write in your letter?

3. How do you write a letter to a physician or psychologist, asking for a financial benefit (or offering a financial benefit) for recommending clients? After all, attorneys specializing in accident and malpractice claims give a portion of their contingency fees to lawyers who refer clients.

4. I want to offer free hearing screenings to the elderly in my community. It will serve the purposes of addressing an unmet need of this population and drawing attention to my audiology practice. Is this ethical? If it is, how do I do it?

5. I can't afford the high registration fees and transportation costs of attending the ASHA or AAA conventions, but I need to get 30 hours of continuing education every 3 years to keep my CCC and my state license. What should I write to ASHA about this?

ANSWERS

1. Although the format of a friendly letter, as opposed to business format, is acceptable when writing to a former professor, the salutation is inappropriate, verging on insulting. The first sentence is aggressive in construction and indicates a lack of respect for the professor by giving only 1 week of notice for the requested letter. The second sentence is actually a relative clause, that is, a sentence fragment. Mr. di Sappoint should have added, "I would be grateful," either before or after the clause. The third sentence is a run-on, and should be ended after the word *director*. The casual tone represented by *thanks* instead of *thank you* reinforces the sense that Mr. di Sappoint will likely disappoint if given the job. Finally, the unethical arm-twisting implied by the requested leverage would almost certainly result in refusal of the recommendation request.

2. You should not apply, and, if invited, you should not go. Scandinavicon would not be abiding by the ASHA Code of Ethics (Principle of Ethics IV) in offering cushy trips in exchange for a hard sell. Even if it is not specifically stated, the implication of a *quid pro quo* (giving something in exchange for something) puts you in ethical hot water.

3. This is a trick question. The ASHA Code of Ethics (Principle of Ethics IV) prohibits you from soliciting, collecting, or even paying these kinds of referral fees.

4. It is ethical (Principle of Ethics III), and ASHA or your state or regional speech, hearing, and language association can help. Visit http://www.asha.org to learn how to prepare a press release, perhaps offering screenings in May to coincide with Better Hearing and Speech Month.

5. All you need to write is http://www.asha.org on your computer search engine. Follow the links to continuing education, and you will find knowledgeable people to assist you. Some of your lower-cost options include completing continuing education (CE) questions in ASHA special interest

group publications, attending colloquia or symposia sponsored by CE providers, or starting your own journal study group, as well as getting credit for teaching a new course or publishing a journal article.

APPENDIX 3A
Sample Institutional Review Board Research Review Form

Date submitted:

TITLE OF PROJECT:

PRINCIPAL INVESTIGATOR/CO-INVESTIGATOR:

Address:

Phone:

E-mail:

You must complete a training program in the protection of human research participants before you can begin your research. Please indicate the date the training was completed and include a copy of the certification with this application.

If you have not completed a training program, follow the links to http://cme.cancer.gov/c01 or http://my.research.umich.edu/peerrs/ or http://www.nyu.edu/ucaihs/tutorial/

I. Brief description of the project's purposes:

II. Planned dates for initiation and completion of the project:

III. Number of subjects:

IV. Characteristics of subjects (e.g., age range, special populations, etc.):

V. Method of subject recruitment:

VI. Brief description of project's methods and research design:

VII. Sequence of activities required of the subject:

VIII. Estimated time commitment required of the subjects:

IX. Any potential risks, discomforts, or stresses and the precautions taken to minimize them:

Signatures and date of all researchers who will be working in direct contact with study participants. These signatures indicate that all the researchers have familiarized themselves with policies regarding the legal and ethical treatment of human subjects in research, and are certified in human subjects protections training.

Name: _____

Date: _____

Signature: _____

Affiliation: _____
                          (institution/organization)

ATTACHMENTS CHECKLIST:

1. Informed Consent Form
2. Debriefing Form (if applicable)
3. Representative sample of materials/test/questionnaire items
4. Sign-up sheet, solicitation script, or advertisement (whichever is applicable)
5. Other attachments

CHAPTER 4

Using Internet Resources

The dot-com boom and bust of the late 1990s into the new century were startling reminders of the blinding speed and mutability of the Internet. Fortunes were won and lost on companies that sometimes appeared to be barely more than dreams. A new English syntax grew in the youth-friendly domains of e-mail and Facebook. Emoticons, such as the colon plus hyphen plus closed parentheses to represent the "smiley-face" (☺) icon, addressed the inherent lack of affect in writing as opposed to speaking. A pair of smart students in California developed a user-friendly means of accessing Internet resources, which led to a new verb form—to Google—and to the former students' new status as billionaires. Search engines replaced trips to the library and bookstore for students writing term papers and clinicians collecting therapy materials. Camera-phones with images and videos later posted on YouTube led to abrupt falls from grace for unprepared and unsuspecting celebrities and politicians.

Welcome to the new way of doing business, meeting your life partner, succeeding in academia, and conducting your clinical practice. There is not much point any more in measuring intelligence by how many things we know, as long as we understand how to access information. Indeed, Guilford's (1967) model of the structure of the intellect should probably be revisited and modified. There is less of a need for convergent behavior, characterized by logical conclusions and logical necessities, when silicone chips can do the hunting and gathering for us. There is more of a need for divergent behavior, characterized by logical alternatives and logical possibilities. We have the time and the nonsilicone abilities of creativity and imagination, which permit original synthesis of the avalanche of information coming through our computers.

What Is the Internet?

The interconnected network of networks is a worldwide collection of cooperating institutions. No corporation, not Microsoft or Google, no government, no university or library, no individual or group of individuals owns all or any part of the Internet (convention is to capitalize the *I*).

A history of the Internet (Leeper & Gotthoffer, 2001) usually begins with the U.S. Defense Department in the mid-1960s, which sought to protect the nation against Cold War enemies. The interstate highway system, recently completed, was to have had an analogy in computing resources, linking information rather than transportation, but the projected cost was prohibitive. The Advanced Research Projects Agency (ARPA) was the funding arm of the Defense Department, having invested large sums in computing hardware, graphics programs, and artificial intelligence. The next project, involving networking, would permit sharing of information, so that computer systems could communicate with each other. The resultant ARPANET was used for preliminary research, the first e-mails, and, inevitably, games.

By the 1980s, a time when young men carried transistor radios the size of photocopy machines on their shoulders, the government had eased out of the Internet in favor of business and institutional applications. An early academic use familiar to one of the authors (RG) was BITNET, developed at the City University of New York (CUNY), which permitted electronic mail and transfer of data between select CUNY centers and other academic institutions. Early transfer of data and e-mails between coauthors in New York and California was exhilarating, leading to a new and more efficient way of doing research with multiple authors and sites. There were similar "Eureka" moments with respect to software. One humanities software application analyzed word usage in literature. After RG dutifully analyzed Alexander Pope's poem, *The Rape of the Lock*, and found that, of the total number of words used, about 70% were not duplicated, it was a short logical step to apply the program to a spontaneous language sample in order to obtain a type-token ratio. The sophistication level of current software is about as far removed in speed and size from the old programs as an iPod is from the old boombox.

Syntax, Semantics, and Jargon

The authors had two problems in writing this section:

1. Most readers will be as familiar with the Internet as members
   of the authors' generations were with the typewriter and
   rotary telephone. Some will adapt with more or less difficulty
   than others to successive generations of electronic advances.
   New generations of scholars are needed about every
   10 years; electronic generations seem to turn over about
   every 5 years.
2. Information provided here may be out of date by the time the
   book goes to print. The authors have attempted to include
   information that is as enduring as possible, but some topics
   may appear dated, even quaint, by the time this book is
   published.

Internet Glossary: An Exercise in Futility

Although some reference terms will likely continue to be useful,
there is no substitute for a personal glossary of Internet terms. As
noted in Chapter 1, most professions develop jargon using abbreviations, acronyms, terms based on other languages, and code words,
and the computer science profession is no exception.

1. *Domain:* The three letters after the dot, of which there are
   six common categories:
   a. com (commercial)
   b. edu (educational)
   c. gov (government)
   d. mil (military)
   e. net (network)
   f. org (organization)
2. *E-mail:* Electronic Internet mailbox. The computer of the
   selected Internet Service Provider represents the post office,
   and the user accesses a mailbox through a combination of
   letters and numbers (password).

3. *FTP:* File Transfer Protocol, which allows the user to send (also called *uploading*) and receive (also called *downloading*) files across the Internet.

4. *http://:* HyperText Transfer Protocol, which identifies the way that the file or document will be transferred. Another version is https:// where the last letter indicates *secure*. The protocol indicates the method that Internet software uses to exchange data with a file server.

5. *Hypertext:* A technology enabling combinations of text, graphics, sound, video, and links on a single www page.

6. *ISP:* Internet Service Provider, or your Internet account. Most students have an account through a college or university or by a commercial provider.

7. *Netiquette:* Net etiquette, of which there are several types:

   a. *Emoticon:* The body language of the Internet, consisting mostly of variations on Smiley, including frowning (☹) and winking (;-)) versions.

   b. *Flame:* To insult, hurt, and offend another user in a debasing message.

   c. *Lurk:* To refrain from immediately posting a message on a newsgroup, in order to become more familiar with the style, tone, and content of the messages.

   d. *SHOUT:* To type in ALL CAPS.

   e. *Spam:* The junk mail of the Internet.

8. *URL:* Universal Resource Locator, which enables the user to locate a Web page. For example, http://www.pluralpublish ing.com is a URL that will connect the user to the publisher of this book. The American Psychological Association (APA, 2001) offers a useful diagram of a URL (Figure 4–1). The host name is often the address for a home page. Test the URL before submitting a paper, because two problems are common:

   a. The URL may be copied incorrectly; or,

   b. The site may have moved.

9. *Username:* Also called userid, account name or number. The authors may be reached at serpanos@adelphi.edu and goldfarb2@adelphi.edu. The numeral in the second username acknowledges that there are two (or more) faculty members with the same name.

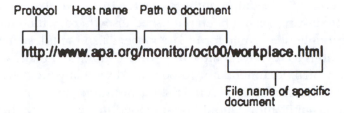

Figure 4–1. Sample URL. From *Publication Manual of the American Psychological Association* (5th ed., p. 270), by the American Psychological Association, 2001, Washington, DC: Author. Retrieved March 2, 2009, from http:www.apastyle.org

10. *Viruses, worms, and Trojan horses:* Dangerous programs designed to perform an undesired task, such as erasing the hard disk, through deception.
11. *www:* The World Wide Web, developed in the 1990s by the European Laboratory for Particle Physics.

Uses and Abuses

Research resources on the Internet may or, more frequently, may not be peer reviewed. Evaluation by a panel of experts before publishing is an accepted process in the scholarly community to reduce error, fraud, and prejudice. Many peer-reviewed professional journals, including those published by ASHA, require electronic submission of articles, and appear on-line as well as in hard copy. A member of the American Speech-Language-Hearing Association (ASHA) or NSSHLA (the student organization) can access peer-reviewed journal articles in electronic form as follows: Go to http://www.asha .org→click on ASHA journals→Login with e-mail address and password→select one of the ASHA Journals Online.

The editor of the *American Journal of Speech-Language Pathology* (AJSLP; Hoit, 2005) addressed some ethical issues that relate to the writing process. She noted that manuscripts available on an individual's Web site are considered published (but not peer reviewed). AJSLP requires authors to state in a cover letter that the submitted work has not been published elsewhere, which includes publication in electronic form. The journal also includes a letter of instructions to reviewers indicating that a submitted manuscript is a confidential document, not to be shared with anyone else.

As a general rule of scholarship, only references from peer-reviewed publications should be included in research reports. For electronic articles or Internet-only journals, find a publisher's statement, such as the following: *The Journal of Speech-Language Pathology and Applied Behavior Analysis* (JSLP-ABA), ISSN: 1932-4731, is published by Joseph Cautilli. It is a peer-reviewed, electronic journal intended for circulation in the scientific community.

Human participants in research, particularly those children and adults with communication disorders, need special protection (Schwartz, 2006). In most types of peer-reviewed published research there are two and often three gatekeepers. The first review, before humans may participate in research, comes from the Institutional Review Board (IRB), which must comply with federal regulations and ethical guidelines set forth in DHHS Regulations US CFR 46, NSF Regulations US CFR 690, and The Belmont Report. The IRB, generally including peers and a volunteer member from the broader community, reviews the proposal or research design as well as completion of required IRB forms. These forms require a description of the project's purposes, methods, and design; initiation and completion dates; characteristics and number of participants; recruitment method; and any potential risks, discomforts, or stresses, and precautions taken to minimize them (Goldfarb, 2006). The second gatekeeper is the funding agency. Although many studies are completed without external funding, many papers in ASHA journals will cite the funding source in the acknowledgments section at the end of the article. For example, recognition of support from NIH means that the National Institutes of Health provided funding, usually in the form of new-investigator support (a number beginning with RO3) or as multiyear major funding (a number beginning with RO1). Grants of any type are very competitive, and funding will be provided only after a careful review, similar to but more stringent than that of the IRB, above. The final gatekeeper is the scholarly journal, which has its own peer-review process, but generally includes an editor and several associate editors with expertise in the topic of the submitted manuscript. Erroneous, fraudulent, and prejudicial papers still occasionally find their way into print, but such an event is so rare as to be newsworthy.

Beginning in 2000, anyone submitting a grant proposal to NIH was (and still is) required to complete a computer-based training course on the protection of human research participants. This free course on research ethics is available (subject to change) at http://www.cme.cancer.gov/c01 or http://ohsr.od.nih.gov or for those who are not employees of NIH, http://cme.cancer.gov/clinicaltrials/learning/humanparticipant-protections.asp. A student who completes the course is permitted to print a certificate of completion. Students and researchers should also visit the Belmont Report Historical Archive at http://www.hhs.gov/ohrp/belmontArchive.html to see interviews with members of the National Commission for the Protection of Human Subjects of Biomedical and Behavioral Research in a 9-minute video. Among other Web sites offering information or tutorials on ethics are the following:

1. Go to the site and click on "Health topics" to learn about ethics and health at http:www.who.int
2. Information on human subject research is available from http://www.cdc.gov. Scroll along the alphabetical listings for a wealth of information.
3. In 1994 President Clinton established the Department of Energy's Advisory Committee on Human Radiation Experiments. Of particular interest is "Part I. Ethics of Human Subjects Research: A Historical Perspective" at http://www.hhs.gov/ohrp/education/index.html#materials .
4. In the National Library of Medicine's "Current Bibliographies in Medicine" there are 500 references in "Ethical Issues in Research Involving Human Participants." The site, including President Clinton's 1997 apology to the survivors of the Tuskegee syphilis study, is at http://www.nlm.nih.gov/archive//20061214/pubs/cbm/hum_exp.html .
5. The "World Medical Association Declaration of Helsinki Ethical Principles for Medical Research Involving Human Subjects," adopted 1964 and amended most recently in October 2000, is at http://www.nihtraining.com/ohsrsite/guidelines/helsinki.html .

Comdisdome (ContentScan) - includes topics in audiology and speech-language pathology, covering journal articles, books, dissertations, grants, websites, and information on relevant authors and institutions. Journal coverage, 1965 to the present, includes citations and abstracts with some full text available.	Database
Communication & Mass Media Complete (Ebscohost) - provides the most robust, quality research solution in areas related to communication and mass media. This database originated with the merging of the CommSearch and Mass Media Articles Index databases.	Full-text database
Education Full Text (Wilson) - indexes and abstracts articles from periodicals and yearbooks. Books relating to education published in 1995 or later are also indexed. Abstracting coverage begins with January 1994. Full-text coverage begins in January 1996.	Full-text database
Eric (CSA) (CSA) - covers conferences, meetings, government documents, theses, dissertations, reports, audiovisual media, bibliographies, directories, books and monographs in the field of Education, from 1966 to the present.	Database
Eric (Ebcohost) (Ebscohost) - citations and abstracts from over 980 educational and education-related journals, as well as full text of more than 2,200 digests.	Full-text database
Eric (Firstsearch) citations for articles in education periodicals and for documents on ERIC microfiche	Database
Eric (Free on the web) the United States Department of Education operates this ERIC database containing more than one million records going back to 1966. More than 100,000 non-journal documents (issued 1993-2004), are available in full-text at no cost.	Full-text database
Linguistics and Language Behavior Abstracts (CSA) - provides abstracts and bibliographical citations from 1973-present in the study and use of language, including topics such as psycholinguistics, special education, nonverbal communication and hearing and speech physiology.	Database
Medline with Full Text (Ebscohost) - provides full text for nearly 1,200 journals indexed in MEDLINE, including more than 1,400,000 full-text articles dating back to 1965.	Full-text database
MedlinePlus (free on the web) - extensive information from the National Institutes of Health and other trusted sources on over 650 diseases and conditions. Includes lists of hospitals and physicians, a medical encyclopedia and dictionary, information on prescription and nonprescription drugs, health information from the media, and links to thousands of clinical trials.	Database

Figure 4–2. Sample database search. From Adelphi University. Retrieved October 14, 2008, from http://libraries/adelphi.edu/journal/databases.php

Now that you have learned some of the history and ethical behavior in conducting research with individuals who have communication disorders, you are ready to use the Internet to study these disorders.

University libraries have access to a variety of databases in specialized areas. Figure 4–2 lists some sites of interest to those undertaking research in audiology and speech-language pathology, based on Adelphi University Library listings.

Citing References from the Internet

For specific style questions that may not be addressed in this section, refer to electronic reference formats recommended by the American Psychological Association. The URL is http://www.apastyle.org/elecref.html.

The variety of material available on the Web, and the variety of ways in which it is structured and presented, can present challenges for creating usable and useful references. Referencing from the Web is challenging. Although both Modern Language Association (MLA) and American Psychological Association (APA) styles are used widely, our professions favor APA style. Following are guidelines for authors using and citing Internet sources, based on APA (2001) style:

1. Direct readers as closely as possible to the information being cited; whenever possible, reference specific documents rather than home or menu pages.
2. Provide references that work.

What kinds of documents are available on the Internet? They may be articles in periodicals (e.g., newspaper, newsletter, or journal); they may stand on their own, not as part of a volume (e.g., research paper, government report, online book or brochure); or they may be uniquely Web based (e.g., Web page, newsgroup). Internet references should include document title or description, date (either the date of publication or update or the date of retrieval), and the URL. Identify the authors of a document when possible.

Following are examples of APA (2001) style for Internet referencing.

Electronic Article

This is the same as for the print version, but if you have viewed the article only in its electronic form, you should add in brackets the phrase "electronic version."

Reference:

> Ambrose, N. G., & Yairi, E. (2002). The Tudor study: Data and ethics. [Electronic version]. *American Journal of Speech-Language Pathology*, *11*, 190–203.

In-text:

> (Ambrose & Yairi, 2002)

Electronic Article (where the format is modified from the print version)

> Author, A. A., Author, B. B., & Author, C. C. (2000). Title of article. *Title of Periodical*, *vol. no.*, year. Retrieved month day, year, from URL.

In-text:

> (Author et al., year)

Specific Internet Document

Reference:

> *Electronic reference formats recommended by the American Psychological Association.* (2001). Retrieved January 2, 2007, from http://www.apastyle.org/elecref.html

In-text:

> (American Psychological Association [APA], 2001)

In-text (subsequent references):

> (APA, 2001)

Article in an Internet-Only Journal

Reference:

> Goldfarb, R. (2006). Operant conditioning and programmed instruction in aphasia rehabilitation. *The Journal of Speech-Language Pathology and Applied Behavior Analysis*, *1*, 56–65. Retrieved January 2, 2007, from http://www.behavior-analyst-today.com/SLP-ABA-VOL-1 /SLP-ABA-1-1.pdf

In-text:

> (Goldfarb, 2006)

Evaluating Internet Sources for Professional Writing

Anyone can post anything on a personal Web site or to a newsgroup. A particularly intriguing, entertaining, or controversial story has the potential to "go viral," a process whereby the posting in the morning circumnavigates the globe during the day and appears on CNN that evening. The extraordinary number of hits on the site, distribution via electronic mailing lists, and downloads can impose a sense of authority or gravitas to the posting. Not all of these postings are frivolous, nefarious, or sexual; some represent the best efforts of well-meaning people. For example, the notion that a preservative used for vaccines had a direct link to the development of autism has circulated the Internet for years. There have been no double-blinded randomized clinical trials (the gold standard of research) in support of a causal relationship between vaccines and autism, but some parents, through fear or lack of adequate critical evaluation, have put their young children at risk by refusing to have them vaccinated against preventable childhood diseases. Indeed, one of our doctoral students, at the beginning of her studies, submitted a research proposal (not accepted by her mentor) based on the vaccine-autism link "proven" in Internet reports.

Following are some strategies for educated consumers of Internet research:

1. Read the URL. As noted above, the host name (e.g., asha.org) tells you the source or sponsor of the site. Be sure of the domain, though. Entering whitehouse.gov will take you to the residence of the U.S. President, but whitehouse.com will take you to a porn site. (Don't try this at home.) If the source is a major newspaper, the Web site should be given the same weight as the print version. If the source is not familiar, search for verifiable data, rather than vague or generic terms, such as "most people" or "leading scientists."
2. Establish a comfort level. Lurk in newsgroups or listservs before posting. Avoid sites where boasts, generalities, and flames are common. Use a search engine to verify the host. Of course, evaluate the style and competence of the writing.

Be aware that the test of comfort is not part of the scientific method (see "Evidence-Based Writing," Chapter 2).

3. Verify, using independent sources. The same information is represented on the Internet via different paths. Newsgroups often skew the information to the direction of their political or cultural agendas, so visit other newsgroups with compatible as well as opposing points of view. Try to follow cited information back to their sources or contact the writer of the posting for reference material. Remember that, just as an author of a book may misunderstand or misrepresent information gleaned from other sources, the person posting in a newsgroup may not be correct in interpreting source material (even more likely, as newsgroup postings do not undergo peer review).

4. Be skeptical. The vastness of the Internet permits topics to be analyzed in fair and balanced or very narrowly focused ways. The nonprejudicial nature of the Internet requires that all Web sites, from megacorporations to garage-level start-ups, be delivered to the end user with the same speed and quality. At present the U. S. Congress is considering a request from several giant corporations to legislate a two-tiered system on the Internet that will favor those businesses that spend more money. We oppose this as scholars who support the ready and equal availability of information of all types. The Internet does not need owners or masters, and it is the job of critical thinkers to separate the wheat from the chaff.

5. Be curious. Following links in Web sites is similar to reading the articles and books listed in the bibliography section of a journal article. In both cases, the reader's own determination to understand original source material may yield information that supports or refutes the author's claims. Either way, the reader will be performing the nonsilicone tasks of original synthesis and divergent thinking.

We have not discussed MUDs (multi-user dimensions), MOOs (multi-user object orienteds), or IRCs (Internet relay chats), because we do not consider them to be useful research venues. Similarly, chat programs such as ICQ ("I seek you") networks and Web-based programs are fine for buddies but not for scholarly pursuits.

Final Note

The anonymity of the Web makes it tempting to think that e-mails and group postings will never be traced back to the sender. There are many people who are awaiting trials, named in lawsuits, or worse, because they were laboring under this misconception. The general rule is to write anything you want, but think long and hard before clicking the "Send" key. To that good advice we would add that you proofread carefully.

References

American Psychological Association. (2001). *Publication manual of the American Psychological Association* (5th ed.). Washington, DC: Author.

Cautilli, J. (Ed.). (2007). *The Journal of Speech-Language Pathology and Applied Behavior Analysis.* Retrieved January 3, 2007, from http://www.slp-aba.net/Pub-Statement.html

Goldfarb, R. (2006). An atheoretical discipline. In R. Goldfarb (Ed.), *Ethics: A case study from fluency* (pp. 117–137). San Diego, CA: Plural.

Guilford, J. P. (1967). The nature of human intelligence. New York: McGraw-Hill.

Hoit, J. (2005). Write right. *American Journal of Speech-Language Pathology, 17,* 171.

Leeper, L. H., & Gotthoffer, D. (2001). *Communication sciences and disorders on the net.* Boston: Allyn & Bacon.

Schwartz. R. G. (2006). Would today's IRB approve the Tudor study? Ethical considerations in conducting research involving children with communication disorders. In R. Goldfarb (Ed.), *Ethics: A case study from fluency* (pp. 83–96). San Diego, CA: Plural.

EXERCISES

1. Which of the following is not a domain (the three letters after the dot)?

    a. com

    b. edu

    c. gov

    d. mil

    e. mon

2. The protocol that identifies the way that the file or document will be transferred is:

    a. FTP

    b. http

    c. e-mail

    d. hypertext

    e. ISP

3. The junk mail of the Internet is called:

    a. emoticon

    b. flame

    c. lurk

    d. shout

    e. spam

4. In the 1990s, the European Laboratory for Particle Physics developed the:

    a. URL

    b. username

    c. viruses

    d. www

    e. Trojan horses

5. What are some strategies for educated consumers of Internet research?

    a. Read the URL.

    b. Establish a comfort level.

    c. Verify, using independent sources.

    d. Be skeptical.

    e. Be curious.

ANSWERS

1. The answer is *e*; there is no domain for mon (money). The other domains—com (commercial), edu (educational), gov (government), and mil (military) do exist on the Internet.

2. The answer is *b*, for HyperText Transfer Protocol. As we noted in this chapter, *FTP* is File Transfer Protocol, which allows the user to send (also called *uploading*) and receive (also called *downloading*) files across the Internet; *e-mail* is the electronic Internet mailbox; *hypertext* is a technology enabling combinations of text, graphics, sound, video, and links on a single www page; and *ISP* is the Internet Service Provider, or your Internet account.

3. The answer is *e*. *Emoticon* refers to the body language of the Internet, consisting mostly of variations on Smiley, including frowning (☹) and winking (;-)) versions. To *flame* is to insult, hurt, and offend another user in a debasing message. To *lurk* is to refrain from immediately posting a message on a newsgroup, in order to become more familiar with the style, tone, and content of the messages. To *SHOUT* is to type in ALL CAPS.

4. The correct answer is *d*, the World Wide Web. *URL* is the Universal Resource Locator, which enables the user to locate a Web page. The *username* is also called userid, an account name or number. *Viruses* refer to dangerous programs designed to perform an undesired task, such as erasing the hard disk, through deception. A *Trojan horse* is a form of a virus.

5. All the above are strategies we recommend.

CHAPTER 5

Using Library Resources

It's hard to imagine a time when printed information couldn't be retrieved by sitting in front of a computer and clicking a button, yet certainly tangible collections of print works have existed (and still do) in storage areas well known as libraries, which date far back over 5000 years to ancient Mesopotamia. Because much printed information typically housed in libraries can also be accessed electronically via the Internet, the reader is referred to Chapter 4, "Using Internet Resources." This chapter, however, will focus mainly on the information and physical services available to the student of communication sciences and disorders in university libraries.

History of the Library

Private "libraries" or collections of written works originated in the Near East and have existed for thousands of years. The practice prospered with the ancient Greeks through their enlightened curiosity in intellectual life and literacy. The concept of a public library surfaced by the 4th century BC (Krasner-Khait, 2001). The first public library in the United States appeared in 1833 in New Hampshire, with hundreds more opened throughout the country following the surge of immigration and the idea of a free public education for all children.

Catering primarily to the needs of the educated—scholars, scientists, teachers—and later to the larger masses, libraries would clearly play a major role in higher education. The first American university library was established in 1638 at Harvard, the oldest American institution of higher learning, with a donation of over

300 books by the Massachusetts clergyman, John Harvard (Shores, 1972). Today there are over 100,000 libraries of all types in the United States including academic, armed forces, corporate, government, law, medical, public, religious, and school libraries (American Library Association, 2009). Although the type of information housed in libraries has changed drastically over the years, from scrolls to cyberspace bytes, the search for knowledge, and a place to store it, will continue throughout the ages, or as long as there are individuals who seek it.

The student in communication sciences and disorders has access to a wealth of information stored in the university's library. Initially a repository for books, the modern university library additionally includes collections of information such as journals, video and audio recordings, microforms, government documents, and electronic resources. Many also have quiet seating areas to which students can retreat for moments of silent reading or study time during breaks from a busy day of classes or clinical work.

Collections

Books

The Library of Congress (LC) classification system is used by most academic libraries in the country to organize and ease search for books. In this system, a distinctive call number is assigned to each book, which allows organization by subject matter with a combination of letters and numbers (Library of Congress, 2007). The books are arranged in alphanumerical order using the call number, which appears (in order from top to bottom) on the book binding:

RC

423

.V45

2006

1. The first letter of the call number represents the subject.
2. The second letter represents a subdivision of that subject.

3. The first set of numbers refers to an area of study within that subdivision.
4. The second set of numbers is a code that represents the author's name, book title, and subject. It should be read as a decimal, e.g., .45.
5. The last number represents the year of publication.

In the example above, R represents *Medicine*, and C is *Internal Medicine, Practice of Medicine.*

Although the electronic age has dramatically decreased the need for printed materials in general, for practical reasons the printed book is still preferred by readers, and libraries still maintain large print collections for their patrons.

Scholarly Journals

A typical form of publication in the medical, scientific, and technological disciplines, and certainly in the communication sciences, is that of the journal-style article. This type of short work, typically of original research, is written in a discrete subject area and became a common form of disseminating scientific information by the end of the 18th century. The journal is a serial publication, usually published by an academic or professional association or press. *Refereed* or *peer-reviewed* journals indicate that the articles were evaluated by a team of scholars assembled by the editor with expertise in that particular subject matter. The peer reviewers assess the quality of the work, such as the content, mechanics of the writing (grammar, spelling, sentence structure, etc.), and accuracy of the citations, and provide their comments to the author and editor. It is the editor who ultimately decides whether the manuscript is rejected or accepted with or without recommended revisions (Budd, 2005).

The first American professional journal in our discipline, *The Voice*, was published from 1879 to 1892 by the clinician Edgar Werner and focused on the topic of speech disorders, specifically on stuttering. Interestingly, it was the National Society for the Study and Correction of Speech Disorders (NSSCSD), an organization preceding the American Speech-Language-Hearing Association (ASHA), that published the first journal by a professional organization of the communication sciences in July 1918, entitled the *American Journal of Speech Disorders and Correction*. ASHA first published the *Journal of Speech Disorders* in March 1936 (Malone, 1999; Paden, 1975).

Today there are hundreds of journals devoted to various issues and topics in our discipline. Most print journals also allow users electronic access to their articles, and many journals now appear in on-line only formats. Journal collections vary by institution as cost and space are considerations for maintaining them, and therefore not all journals in a specific field may be carried by an academic library. Because libraries must pay journal subscription fees and at the same time adhere to budget restrictions, journal collections are carefully evaluated and periodically reassessed. Print journals are usually arranged on stacked shelving in alphabetical order by title. These take up physical space that may also restrict the holdings, although the wide availability of electronic formats has made space less of an issue.

Audio-Visual Materials

In addition to print media, many informational and instructional materials are available in audio-visual format, including audio cassette or compact disc (CD) recordings; video films, tapes, or digital video discs (DVDs); and electronic software. Instructors may put such items, often limited in number, on reserve to supplement lecture topics. Depending on the specific library policy, the student may have limited access to these materials on-site or with borrowing privileges.

Microforms

Before the wide availability of computers and electronic versions of print documents, librarians found other ways to contend with the growing problem of space. Printed materials, typically books and newspapers, were transferred onto minutely small nonprint media in the form of film, collectively known as microforms. Common types found in libraries include *microfilm*, which refers to 35 mm film wound onto open reels or inserted into cassettes, and *micro-*

fiche, which is a flat piece of film typically stored in filing envelopes. As microforms are reproduced into smaller photographic film images, they then require special magnifying machines for viewing, which can be cumbersome and time consuming to the user. Print copies of the images can be made, but they are often of inferior quality. Because they are analog media, an additional problem with microforms is that they are susceptible to deterioration (Veaner, 2002). Hooray for the digital era!

Services

The Organization of Information: Catalogs and Databases

In order to search effectively for information on a given subject, there must be a systematic method for organization, storage, and retrieval of that information. *Catalogs*, or lists of a library's holdings, were in early centuries simple handwritten registers, usually alphabetized, of the books contained within. Indeed, the library catalog can be considered "the oldest type of booklist known" (Vickery, 1970, p. 20). Such lists were simple to prepare and maintain as long as the collection itself, and interest in it, were minimal. Catalogs were prepared by individuals at separate libraries without a universal system, and therefore varied greatly in organization and quality up until the 19th century. One can only imagine the hours of intensive labor put into hand-writing or manually typing such lists (and periodically updating them) prior to the advent of computers. Over the years various classification schemes emerged in an effort to simplify the task of book searches and retrieval. Contemporary American librarianship began in 1876 with the formation of a professional organization, the American Library Association (ALA), and attempts toward a more systematic approach to cataloging. During the 20th century, the LC advanced the practice of shared cataloging among libraries. The ALA is currently the largest and oldest library organization in the world, providing library and information services, standards for the profession and professional services, and publications to members and the public (ALA, 2007). A division of the ALA, the Association of College and Research Libraries (ACRL), is concerned with aspects of the academic library (ALA, 2004).

With the electronic age came the ability to organize and store vast amounts of cataloged information digitally into *databases* that allowed for easier sharing of this information among libraries and organizations, and for on-line search and retrieval of materials (Blake, 2002; Shoffner, 2002). The use of electronic catalogs was nearly universal in academic libraries by the year 2000 (U.S. Department of Education, 2005). Databases may be isolated to book or journal listings within a single institution, or may be so expansive as to include all types of materials in libraries throughout the world, such as WorldCat, a catalog supported by the Online Computer Library Center (OCLC) and serving over 57,000 libraries in over 100 countries and territories (OCLC, 2007). University library catalogs are available to students on-site or via remote (from outside the university) access. In addition, the library may provide access to a variety of other electronic catalogs or databases such as those of neighboring public or other university libraries as well as state, organizational, or international systems, through the academic library. Though the library is required to pay a site license fee for the use of most databases, in general access to library databases is free of charge to students as part of their library privileges at their academic institution.

A valuable database for students and professionals in the communication sciences is PubMed, a free service developed by the National Center for Biotechnology Information (NCBI) and provided by the U.S. National Library of Medicine and the National Institutes of Health. PubMed encompasses over 17 million citations from the biomedical and life science literature (dentistry, medicine, nursing, veterinary medicine, the health care system, and the preclinical sciences) published worldwide, and includes MEDLINE, its largest database component (NCBI, 2007). There are even databases dedicated solely to reference sources within our field. One such database, ComDisDome (published by ContentScan Inc.), focuses on information sources from the hundreds of books, refereed journals, dissertations, grants, and other related published documents exclusive to the communication sciences and disorders (ContentScan, 2007). An advantage of a discipline-specific database may be that searches often yield more precise and relevant citations to the search topic than when conducted with cross-disciplinary systems such as PubMed. On the other hand, such searches may be limited to the narrower source base of the discipline-specific database. The student must, of course, consider these issues when conducting a search. These text-based databases provide citations and may permit access, with or without charge, to abstracts and full-text articles at journal Web sites or through the library holdings (depending on journal subscription and library site license status) and other related Web resources.

Conducting a Search

Search and you shall find. Today, electronic databases are used to search and access the information in a library's holdings (and beyond) literally in seconds. Most library catalog searches are initiated by typing in a specific piece of information such as a keyword, subject heading, title, author, or catalog number. The databases may also be searched using other numbers including non-LC call numbers, Government Document numbers, ISBN (International Standard Book Number), or ISSN (International Standard Serial Number).

Figure 5–1 is a sample library catalogue database search.

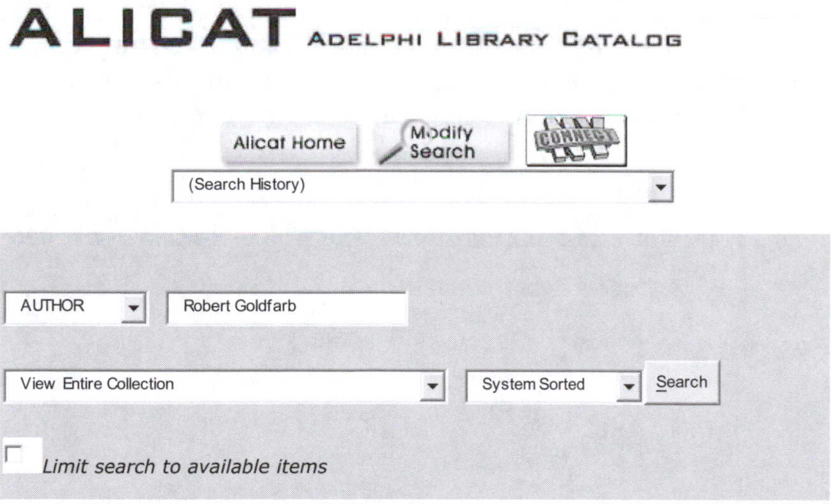

Figure 5–1. Sample library catalog database search. From Adelphi University Libraries. Available at http://allicat.adelphi.edu/. Copyright © 2007 Adelphi University Libraries. All rights reserved. Powered by Innovative Interfaces, Inc. 2007.

Once processed, the result screen will display whether the item is available for circulation or accessible electronically. Books will be identified by call number and a location for retrieval will be provided (see example in Figure 5–2). An option may also be given to place a hold on the item. Journal listings will include the specific volumes owned by the library and whether they are in print or electronic form.

Figure 5–3 is an example of a cross-disciplinary database search by topic (citations excluded). In the example, 1807 articles were found for the topic of sudden deafness using a cross-disciplinary database. A similar search on a disciplinary-specific database system produced 1341 results, a smaller number, but still an inordinate amount to sift through. It is therefore wise to narrow the search as much as possible by typing in as many key words that are relative to the topic as possible. For example, limiting the topic to sudden deafness *in children* produced 239 and 3 citations using the same databases above, respectively, a considerably more manageable outcome.

Interlibrary Loans/Reciprocal Library Privileges

It is very possible that a specific journal or book the student requires is not available through the student's academic library, a problem to which there are solutions. Many universities have reciprocal library

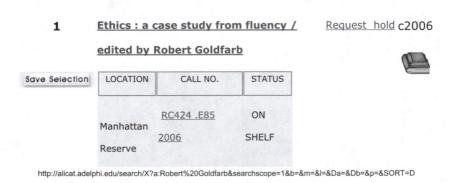

Figure 5–2. Sample catalog search. Available at http://alicat.adelphi.edu/search/X?a:Robert%20Goldfarb&searchscope=1&b=&m=&l=&Da=&Db=&p=&SORT=D.

Pub Med
www.pubmed.gov

A service of the National Library of Medicine
and the National Institutes of Health

| Limits | Preview/Index | History | Clipboard | Details |

Search [PubMed ▼] for [sudden deafness]   GoClear Save Search

| Limits | Preview/Index | History | Clipboard | Details |

All: 1807

http://www.ncbi.nlm.nih.gov/sites/entrez (search conducted July 12, 2007)

Figure 5–3. Sample cross-disciplinary database search by topic (citations excluded). Retrieved July 12, 2007, from http://www.ncbi .nlm.nih.gov/sites/entrez.

privileges with local universities or libraries. Students may use or borrow materials available for circulation, and may access library services. When materials are not owned by the academic library or accessible through its reciprocal databases, a student may request an interlibrary loan electronically or in person at the reference or help desk. Depending on the item, interlibrary loans may take from a few days to weeks to be delivered, so the student should plan accordingly, especially if the item is required for an assignment with a rapidly approaching due date.

Reference Services

Librarians

With the digital age and anonymity of computer use, one may forget that the library does offer opportunities to connect (either electronically or in person) with an expert who is specially trained to work with individuals on researching a particular topic or locating material. In fact, most large academic libraries employ numerous staff members, each with a unique role in the coordination, organization, and management of services. Reference librarians with expertise in a specific subject area are typically hired by the university to serve as liaisons to academic departments. It would, therefore, be particularly useful to the student who is working on a research paper to seek out the library liaison for communication sciences and disorders. Most academic institutions arrange library tours and instructional sessions for their students to gain familiarity with the physical location of materials and services within, including demonstration on performing searches and using catalogs and databases. It should not be forgotten, however, that a student has the option of arranging a one-on-one appointment with the librarian, an opportunity that should definitely be taken (Brophy, 2005; Guerrero, 2006).

Reference Tools

The university library will provide the student with on-site or remote electronic access to numerous reference tools such as dictionaries, encyclopedias, thesauruses, and citation and writing style manuals. A common citation and writing format used by our discipline is that of the American Psychological Association, or "APA style," which is readily available for reference use.

Research Guides

Printed or downloadable versions of guides for writing and research have been prepared by academic libraries for student use. Such "how-to" guides are extremely useful for the independent student who needs some help with preparing a research paper, with information ranging from searching and evaluating sources to properly documenting them. Some topics may include information and tips for:

1. Using library databases and catalogs
2. Remote access to library databases
3. Identifying scholarly vs. popular journals
4. Research and writing
5. Plagiarism
6. Documenting scientific writing
7. Web evaluation

Reserve Items

The library permits faculty to put items that are recommended or required for courses such as books, journal articles, or audio-visual materials aside or *on reserve* for student use. Electronic reserve items are known as *e-reserves*. This service ensures that materials that may be difficult to acquire (such as those limited in number or not typically available in the library collection) are readily available to students. Access to physical reserve items requires a visit to the library service desk and is often time-restricted, usually limiting the user to a few hours or days. More conveniently, e-reserves can be electronically downloaded by the student, as long as there is access to a computer with Internet connection. Students may consider asking the instructor to make use of the reserve service when recommended or required course materials are difficult to obtain.

Course Packs

Many instructors recommend or require reading assignments from sources other than the designated textbook for the course (e.g., journal articles and individual book chapters from other texts). Following copyright approval, photocopies of these reading materials are collected and bound in book form known as a *course pack*, and are prepared as a matter of convenience for students. Course packs are particularly handy when there are numerous readings or when items are difficult to locate (e.g., out of print, not available in the university library). The instructor provides the titles or photocopies of the materials, which are then prepared into course pack form by the university library, printing office, or other service area. Course packs may be provided to students for free as handouts, or sold for a fee through the university bookstore or by the instructor.

Copyright Material

The term *copyright* refers to the legal rights and protection given to authors of their published or unpublished literary or artistic work as provided by the U.S. Constitution and federal law (*Title 17*, U.S. Code). Copyright protection is automatic once the work is created and does not need to be officially registered, though many authors choose to do so in order to obtain a public record or certificate of the registration and eligibility for additional legal and monetary rights (U.S. Copyright Office, 2008). The student should assume, unless it is made known otherwise, that all materials housed in the library that are electronically accessed and that occur in any other forms of information obtained elsewhere are copyrighted. This generally means that reproductions of such materials can be made only with the permission of the copyright holder; however, there are exceptions.

The 1976 Copyright Act delineated the "fair use" modification to copyright violation (or infringement) by allowing limited copies to be made for noncommercial purposes such as for personal study, research, scholarship, or teaching. Therefore, an individual may legally reproduce material under this premise, but could be found liable for copyright violation if at a later time the material is used for purposes beyond fair use. Academic libraries are also, under specific conditions, granted the authority to reproduce materials within the institution itself or for others, but may deny a copy order if it is deemed potentially a copyright infringement. Consider the following distinction. A student is permitted to photocopy a journal article for the purpose of a reading assignment for class. If that student decides, however, to make multiple copies of that article for the purpose of sale to classmates, that would be considered in excess of fair use and that student would be in violation of the copyright law.

Copyright issues have arisen in academic libraries over recent years with the availability of such services as e-reserves and course packs (discussed above) that may infringe on copyright laws, depending on the number and type of items used without author permission. Academic libraries now have guidelines for instructors who use those services in an effort to ensure compliance with the free-use criteria.

Plagiarism

The term *plagiarism* refers to the act of using another's work (ideational, written, or spoken) and intentionally or unintentionally misrepresenting it as one's own. This is essentially considered a form of academic dishonesty or "cheating" by most universities, for which there may be significant repercussions in the academic standing of a student. University students must be especially aware of what constitutes plagiarism, because writing is a major part of academic study. The issue of plagiarism has become more pervasive among institutions over the past years as a result of the widespread use of the Internet by individuals and specifically in academe. Virtually any piece of information on any topic can be found electronically and downloaded rapidly. The ability to access a completed research paper on-line or to find information on a Web page without an obvious author may make it very enticing for one to "borrow" the information. Just as easily, however, instructors have access to search engines specifically geared to finding possible instances of plagiarism, making the offense quickly identifiable.

Certainly, copying another's writing exactly without quotations and reference to the author is an obvious form of plagiarism. However, there are other forms that are not as apparent, leading the student to plagiarize inadvertently. Rewording or paraphrasing the words of someone else without credit to the author is another type of plagiarism. Further, writing ideas that are not one's own without reference to the originator of those ideas is also plagiarism. A simple rule of thumb would be always to provide a reference for the source of information used. The best defense against plagiarism is for the student to be well informed on the subject, and there are numerous sources from which to obtain this information. Most universities have prepared guidelines on plagiarism that are easily available to students through the university library, through a writing center, or electronically. Publication manuals such as the *American Psychological Association Publication Manual* (2001) provide examples of properly referencing and writing citations, and are important resources for the student.

Finally, we counsel sensitivity in dealing with cultures whose custom of honoring ancestors extends to copying what they wrote.

Citing References from Print Books and Journals

In APA format, the references used for the content of a publication are cited in the body of the text by author(s) and date, and also appear in an alphabetical listing in the References section toward the end of the work. The writer must ensure that there is agreement between the references cited in the text and those listed in the References section.

Following are most common uses of APA (2001) style for referencing books and journal articles. The list is not exhaustive, and therefore the reader is referred to the APA style manual for further examples.

Journal Article (One Author)

Reference:

> Serpanos, Y. C. (2004). ABR and DPOAE indices of normal loudness in children and adults. *Journal of the American Academy of Audiology, 15*(8), 555–565.

Notes:

1. The title of the journal article is in sentence case; the journal title is in title case.
2. Journal title and volume are italicized.
3. The journal volume number is added in brackets only if the journal is paginated by issue.

In-text:

> xxxxx xxxxx (Serpanos, 2004)
>
> Serpanos (2004) xxxxx xxxxx

Journal Article (Two Authors)

Reference:

> Serpanos, Y. C., & Jarmel, F. (2007). Quantitative and qualitative follow-up outcomes from a preschool audiologic screening program: Perspectives over a decade. *American Journal of Audiology, 16*, 4–12.

Note: The first word following the colon in the title of a journal article is also capitalized.

In-text:

> xxxxx xxxxx (Serpanos & Jarmel, 2007)
>
> Serpanos and Jarmel (2007) xxxxx xxxxx

Journal Article (Three to Five Authors)

Reference:

> Halpern, H., Goldfarb, R., Brandon, J. M., & McCartin-Clark, M. (1985). Word-association responses to time-altered stimuli by schizophrenic adults. *Perceptual and Motor Skills, 61,* 239–253.

In-text:

> xxxxx xxxxx (Halpern, Goldfarb, Brandon, & McCartin-Clark, 1985)

> Halpern, Goldfarb, Brandon, and McCartin-Clark (1985) xxxxx xxxxx

Note: In works with three to five authors, all author names should be cited the first time the reference is used in the text.

In-text (subsequent references):

> xxxxx xxxxx (Halpern et al., 1985)

> Halpern et al. (1985) xxxxx xxxxx

Note: In subsequent references the surname of the first author is followed by the term *et al.*

Journal Article (Six or More Authors)

Reference:

> Gravel, J., Berg, A., Bradley, M., Cacace, A., Campbell, D., Dalzell, L., et al. (2000). New York State universal new-born hearing screening demonstration project: Effects of screening protocol on inpatient outcome measures. *Ear and Hearing, 21*(2), 131–140.

Note: In journal articles with six or more authors, provide the surnames and initials of the first six authors followed by et al. in the reference list.

In-text:

>xxxxx xxxxx (Gravel et al., 2000)

>Gravel et al. (2000) xxxxx xxxxx

Note: Only the surname of the first author is used followed by the term *et al.* the first and subsequent times the reference is cited in the text.

Entire Book

Reference:

>Raphael, L. J., Borden, G. J., & Harris, K. S. (2007). *Speech science primer: Physiology, acoustics, and perception of speech* (5th ed.). Baltimore, MD: Lippincott, Williams & Wilkins.

Notes:

1. The book title is in sentence case and italicized.
2. A book edition is denoted by the edition number followed by *ed.* in brackets after the book title. The city and state are listed for publishers in the United States and the city, state, and country are listed for those outside the United States; the state or country of publishers in major cities may be omitted: e.g., Baltimore: Lippincott, Williams & Wilkins.

In-text:

>xxxxx xxxxx (Raphael, Borden, & Harris, 2007)

>Raphael, Borden, and Harris (2007) xxxxx xxxxx

Note: Follow rules for citing multiple authors in book references as described in the journal article citation section.

Edited Book

Reference:

>Goldfarb, R. (Ed.). (2006). *Ethics: A case study from fluency*. San Diego, CA: Plural.

Note: Use (Eds.) if there is more than one editor.

In-text:

> xxxxx xxxxx (Goldfarb, 2006)
>
> Goldfarb (2006) xxxxx xxxxx

Chapter in an Edited Book

Reference:

> Goldfarb, R., & Halpern, H. (1989). Impairments of naming and word finding. In C. Code (Ed.), *The characteristics of aphasia* (pp. 33–52). London: Taylor and Francis.

Notes:

1. Both the journal article and book title are in sentence case; the book title is italicized.
2. A frequent error of citation occurs when the editor of a book is listed as the author, but the relevant chapter was written by someone other than the editor. The reference in text would be Goldfarb and Halpern, not Code.

In-text:

> xxxxx xxxxx (Goldfarb & Halpern, 1989)
>
> Goldfarb and Halpern (1989) xxxxx xxxxx

Quoted Material

Reference:
Follow the examples above for referencing journal articles, books, and portions of books.

In-text:

> "xxxxx xxxxx" (Goldfarb & Halpern, 1989, p. 35)
>
> Goldfarb and Halpern (1989) xxxxx "xxxxx xxxxx" (p. 35)

Note: When directly quoting material from another source, the word-for-word section is enclosed within double quotation marks in the body of the text with the author's name, year of publication, and page number of the specific section quoted.

Unpublished Paper Presented at a Professional Meeting

Reference:

> Goldfarb, R., & Bekker, N. (2006, April). *Grammatical category ambiguity in aging, aphasia, and schizophrenia.* Paper presented at the annual meeting of the New York State Speech, Language, and Hearing Association, Saratoga, NY.

Notes:

1. The month of the date of the presentation follows the year by a comma in parentheses.
2. The title of the presentation is in italicized sentence case.
3. Indicate if the professional meeting is annual.
4. Follow the title of the meeting with a comma, then with the city and state abbreviation.

In-text:

> xxxxx xxxxx (Goldfarb & Bekker, 2006)

> Goldfarb and Bekker (2006) xxxxx xxxxx

Poster Session Presented at a Professional Meeting

Reference:

> Schoepflin, J., & Serpanos, Y. (2007, April). *Frequent music listeners: Listening levels and hearing.* Poster session presented at the annual meeting of the American Academy of Audiology, Denver, CO.

In-text:

xxxxx xxxxx (Schoepflin & Serpanos, 2007)

Schoepflin and Serpanos (2007) xxxxx xxxxx

References

American Library Association. (2004). Standards for libraries in higher education. Document ID: 170127. Retrieved March 1, 2009, from http://www.ala.org/ala/mgrps/divs/acrl/standards/standardslibraries.cfm

American Library Association. (2009). Number of libraries in the United States. Retrieved March 1, 2009, from http://www.ala.org/ala/aboutala/hqops/library/libraryfactsheet/alalibraryfactsheet1.cfm

American Psychological Association. (2001). *Publication manual of the American Psychological Association* (5th ed.). Washington, DC: Author.

Blake, V. L. P. (2002). Forging the Anglo-American Cataloging Alliance: Descriptive cataloging, 1830–1908. In M. D. Joachim (Ed.), *Historical aspects of cataloging and classification* (pp. 3–22). Binghamton, NY: The Haworth Information Press.

Brophy, P. (2005). *The academic library.* London: Facet.

Budd, J. M. (2005). *The changing academic library: Operations, culture, environments*. Chicago: Association of College and Research Libraries.

ContentScan Inc. (2007). About the Dome. Retrieved July 11, 2007, from http://www.contentscan.com/dome_about.htm

Guerrero, T. S. (2006). What they don't teach you in library school: Experience is the real teacher. In E. Connor (Ed.), *An introduction to reference services in academic libraries* (pp. 61–76). Binghamton, NY: The Haworth Information Press.

Krasner-Khait, B. (2001). Survivor: The history of the library. *History Magazine, 3*, 47–51.

Library of Congress. (2007). Library of Congress classification outline. Retrieved August 13, 2007, from http://www.loc.gov/catdir/cpso/lcco/

Malone, R. (1999). The first 75 years: An oral history of the American Speech-Language-Hearing Association. Washington, DC: American Speech-Language-Hearing Association.

National Center for Biotechnology Information. (2007). PubMed introduction. Retrieved July 11, 2007, from http://www.ncbi.nlm.nih.gov/entrez/query/static/overview.html#Introduction

Online Computer Library Center. (2007). About OCLC: Furthering access to the world's information. Retrieved June 27, 2007, from http://www.oclc.org/about/default.htm

Paden, E. P. (1975). ASHA in retrospect. Fiftieth anniversary reflections. *ASHA, 17*(9), 571–572.

Shoffner, R. M. (2002). Appearance and growth of computer and electronic products in libraries. In R. E. Abel (Ed.), *Scholarly publishing: Books, journals, publishers, and libraries in the twentieth century* (pp. 209–256). New York: Wiley.

Shores, L. (1972). *Origins of the American college library*. Boston: Gregg Press.

U.S. Copyright Office, Library of Congress. (2008). Copyright office basics. Retrieved March 1, 2009, from http://www.copyright.gov/circs/circ1.pdf

U.S. Department of Education, National Center for Education Statistics. (2005). *The condition of education 2005*, NCES 2005-094, Washington, DC: U.S. Government Printing Office.

Veaner, A. B. (2002). From bibliotheque to omnitheque. In R. E. Abel (Ed.), *Scholarly publishing: Books, journals, publishers, and libraries in the twentieth century* (pp. 163–177). New York: Wiley.

Vickery, B. C. (1970). *Techniques of information retrieval.* Hamden, CT: Archon Books.

EXERCISES

1. In the following alphanumeric display of the Library of
   Congress classification system, which is NOT true?

   RC
   423
   .V45
   2006

   a. The first letter of the call number represents the subject.
   b. The second letter represents the object.
   c. The first set of numbers refers to an area of study within
      that subdivision.
   d. The second set of numbers is a code that represents the
      author's name, book title, and subject. It should be read as
      a decimal, e.g., .45.
   e. The last number represents the year of publication.

2. *Refereed* or *peer-reviewed* journals indicate that:

   a. The articles were evaluated by a team of scholars
      assembled by the editor with expertise in that particular
      subject matter.
   b. Peer reviewers assessed the content of the work, but not
      the mechanics of the writing (grammar, spelling, sentence
      structure, etc.).
   c. The citations were in APA style.
   d. Peer reviewers ultimately decide whether the manuscript
      is rejected or accepted with or without recommended
      revisions.
   e. The journal is published quarterly (four times a year).

3. The largest and oldest library organization in the world
   is the:

   a. Library of Congress
   b. Association of College and Research Libraries (ACRL)
   c. British Museum
   d. American Library Association (ALA)
   e. Google

4. A database dedicated solely to reference sources within our field is:

    a. PubMed
    b. Science Direct
    c. MEDLINE
    d. NIH
    e. ComDisDome

5. On-site or remote electronic access to numerous reference tools such as dictionaries, encyclopedias, thesauruses, and citation and writing style manuals can also be called:

    a. reference librarians
    b. course packs
    c. reference tools
    d. research guides
    e. reserve items

ANSWERS

1. The answer is *b*. The second letter represents a subdivision of that subject.

2. The answer is *a*. Peer reviewers assess both content and mechanics of the writing. Citation style depends on the journal. The journal editor makes the ultimate decisions about acceptance or rejection, but generally follows the advice of the peer reviewers. Finally, different journals have different publication schedules.

3. The answer is *d*. The Library of Congress advanced the practice of shared cataloging among libraries, but is not the largest library organization. The ACRL is a division of ALA, devoted to academic libraries. The British Museum houses the Rosetta Stone and other treasures, but it is not the largest library organization. Finally, Google has expressed the goal of digitizing all library holdings, but has not yet come close to realizing that goal.

4. The answer is *e*. PubMed is a free service developed by the National Center for Biotechnology Information (NCBI). Science Direct publishes electronic versions of journals in our field, such as *Brain and Language* and the *Journal of Communication Disorders*, as well as many other journals in related fields. MEDLINE is the largest database component of PubMed. Finally, the National Institutes of Health (NIH) is a very important federal agency, but it is not a database.

5. The answer is *c*. A number of reference librarians with expertise in a specific subject area are typically hired by the university to serve as liaisons to academic departments. Photocopies of reading materials collected and bound in book form are known as a *course pack*, and are prepared as a matter of convenience for students. Printed or downloadable versions of guides for writing and research have been prepared by academic libraries for student use. Finally, the library permits faculty to put items that are recommended or required for courses such as books, journal articles, or audio-visual materials aside or on reserve for student use. Electronic reserve items are known as *e-reserves*.

CHAPTER 6

Writing for Oral Presentation

In an "On Language" column in the *Chicago Tribune* on November 8, 2006, Nathan Bierma related an anecdote about a visiting professor giving a speech at Columbia University. The speaker reported that two negatives often make a positive, but no language used two positives to make a negative. Another professor in the audience shot back, "Yeah, yeah."

Oral presentations fall into four methods of delivery: impromptu, memorized, manuscript, and extemporaneous. With the exception of the impromptu or spontaneous speech, oral presentations do require some level of preparation in a written form of the speech and in practice of the delivery. A memorized delivery is one where the speech has been committed to memory from a prepared script, and the manuscript delivery is one that is read word for word. The extemporaneous method, the most common form used in classrooms and general public speaking, is a combination of the three styles where notes or an outline are used with a high level of spontaneity in the delivery (Seiler & Beall, 1999). Since it is probable the student of communication sciences will use this format in presentations conducted in the classroom, clinical setting, or professional conferences, this chapter will focus on strategies in the written preparation and execution of an extemporaneous style of oral presentation.

Preparing the Oral Presentation

In any effective oral presentation except the impromptu style, some level of research, writing, and preparation of the delivery is required. The extent of the research, writing, and preparation depends on various factors such as the speaker's style, comfort with and knowledge of the content, and the length and depth of the presentation itself.

Knowledge of a particular topic is required in order for anyone to be able to speak comfortably and convincingly to an audience. The first step in preparing the presentation is to determine how much information needs to be gathered, which is dependent upon the speaker's expertise or knowledge on the specific topic. The research involved in oral presentation should follow the same guidelines used in writing a research paper. Statements made by the speaker should be supported by facts either stated in the presentation or in a printed reference list. In other words, orally presented information is bound by the same principles of ethics and plagiarism as the written form (see Chapter 2: Evidence-Based Writing; Chapter 3: Ethics of Professional Writing; and Chapter 5: Using Library Resources).

Developing the Speech

Though topics vary widely, there is a uniform organization and precise order of the components in all speeches—the introduction, body, and conclusion. A proper speech must follow this sequence; however, this is not necessarily the order in which you will prepare it. Once you have identified the topic, the next step is to create a *statement of purpose*, which will clarify the objective of the speech or the information the audience should receive. The purpose statement also helps to give focus to the development of the talk. Before you begin writing, it is necessary to know the level of familiarity your audience has with the topic and plan the information to be presented accordingly. For example, if the audience has little or no knowledge of the topic, the speaker may need to spend time providing definitions or modifying technical language so that it is readily understood. Alternatively, if the audience presents with a specific level of knowledge of the topic, it would be wasting time, and possibly insulting, to define or explain professional terms.

To write the body of the speech it is necessary to identify the *main points*, or major subdivisions, and organize them in a logical sequence. There may be subpoints to the main ones, and there must be support provided for each main point, which is essentially the "filling" of the speech. Forms of support may be reported by the speaker by providing examples, references, or statistics, presented visually by tables, figures, or other images, or in audio-video format. It is helpful first to organize the main points, subpoints, and supporting points in the form of an outline (see below).

Once the body of the speech has been created, the introduction should be written. Depending on the nature of the presentation and whether there are preceding introductory remarks given by another, the introduction serves to direct the audience to the topic, relate the main points, and motivate listening. The introduction should be brief and should set the tone for what is to come. For reasons similar in importance to making a good first impression, experienced speakers attempt to create an attention-grabbing start. Several strategies may be used to stimulate listeners, such as presenting an analogy, question, quotation, or statement, or humor in the form of a short story or joke. It is important to note that not all work on every occasion, and an introduction must be chosen carefully so that it is appropriate to the nature of the topic, composition of the audience, and comfort level of the speaker.

Finally, the conclusion of the presentation should be prepared. The goal is to end the talk by concisely summarizing the main points as reinforcement of the message and providing final thoughts or suggestions. New information should not be added in this section. Similar to the introduction, the strategies for gaining audience attention may also be used in ending remarks.

Outlining the Presentation

Using an outline for the speech is helpful in two ways. First, the outline is used in the development stage to help the speaker organize the body of the speech. This outline, using complete sentences, serves to define the main, sub-, and supporting points and assists the writer in keeping on track with the topic. Additionally, during the presentation the complete sentence outline can be reduced to a *topic outline* using key words or phrases, which can serve as a visual display to guide the speaker and the audience through the speech.

A common outline style is known as the Harvard outline format, which alternates indented numbers with letters to distinguish main points from supporting points (as many as needed), with at least two at each level (O'Hair, Friedrich, Wiemann, & Wiemann, 1997). From general to specific, the outline uses uppercase Roman numerals, followed by indented capital letters, Arabic numbers, lowercase letters, and lowercase Roman numerals. This style is based on the idea that breaking something results in at least two pieces. For example, supporting a main point requires that there be at least two subpoints, as follows:

  I. First main point
    A. First subpoint
      1. First support point
        a. First sub-support point
          i. First sub-sub-support point
         ii. Second sub-sub-support point
        b. Second sub-support point
      2. Second support point
    B. Second subpoint
  II. Second main point

Once the speech has been written in its entirety, a speaker may find it additionally helpful to create a *speaker's outline*, by writing key words and phrases onto index cards that can be referred to during the speech. The goal of writing the speech is to allow you to set out the complete points of information that you wish to convey. Your goal should be not to read the speech word for word, but to know it so well that you can relay it by referring to abbreviated segments projected on screen or printed onto notes.

Delivering the Oral Presentation

Computer-Generated Presentations

Visual aids such as graphics in the form of charts, diagrams, graphs, photographs, or tables, tangible items such as objects or models, and text are extremely effective in strengthening an oral presentation. Research indicates that information presented orally together with visual support is retained longer by listeners (Zayas-Baya, 1977). Today, with the wide acceptance and availability of computers in personal, educational, and professional use, the computer-generated presentation (a visual counterpart to the speech) is recognized as a standard presentational form.

In this type of presentation, computer-generated or imported images or text are arranged onto individual slides of information created onto a background selected from a variety of color and layout schemes, which are saved into a file. Additionally, audio and video clips can be downloaded from cameras, movies, or other multimedia to be incorporated into the slides. Several software programs are available that provide users with the tools to create computer-generated presentations, the most popular of which is PowerPoint (by Microsoft Corporation).

The visual presentation uses a computer interfaced with a video projector to display the slides of information on a screen viewed by the audience and is typically accompanied by an oral narration. A handout of the presentation slides can also be provided, giving listeners a tangible, additional visual aid to follow and take notes on during the presentation. For a PowerPoint handout, we recommend using a layout of three slides on the left side of the page, with lines for note-taking on the right side.

Creating Computer-Generated Presentations

Among the more frustrating experiences for students, as well as graduates attending professional presentations, is the computer-generated presentation characterized by:

1. the presenter reading the slides to you;
2. slides with so much information that you can't focus on what the presenter is saying, much less get through it all before it clicks ahead;
3. images or text that are not clearly or easily seen from far seating;
4. "bells and whistles" in the form of animation and sound effects that fail to mask a presentation devoid of content or interest, or so many effects that they distract attention from the speaker.

Here are a few rules for preparing your computer-generated presentation (Grice & Skinner, 1998; Miculka, 1999; Treholm, 1999; Zarefsky, 2002):

1. Use color to contrast the slide background with text to make the slides interesting, or to add emphasis by highlighting key sections of text or images. Keep the color schemes and background layout similar throughout the presentation for uniformity and keep it simple; too much color can create a busy-looking slide.
2. Refer to the information on the slide, but never read it to your audience.
3. Try for a limit of seven words per line and seven lines per slide; use bulleted sentences or phrases to separate thoughts.
4. Verify that images are not distorted when enlarged and that graphs or tables are clearly labeled. Use basic fonts (avoid using "fancy" fonts such as script or decorative types or all capitalized letters in text, as they are visually more difficult to read) and large font sizes for text to ensure visibility from a distance, e.g., title: 44 point type, subtitle: 32 point type, text: 28 point type.
5. Use pictures, cartoons, jokes, racing car noises, and other "enhancements" sparingly, so that their effect will be magnified when you do use them. Remember that animation and sound may not work on a computer with a different operating system than the one you used to program your presentation, so plan accordingly. Make sure to reference all copied or downloaded materials.

Factors in Effective Speech Delivery

In addition to thorough content and knowledge of the topic, vocal and physical characteristics and self-confidence in the speaker will affect audience attention, interest, and perception of the speaker's credibility, and therefore must be considered for an effective speech delivery.

Listeners will judge the *quality* of the speaker's voice in terms of tone (e.g., nasal, harsh, melodic, etc.) and manner (arrogant, bored, excited). Speaking with enthusiasm is contagious; if you radiate energy, your audience will likely be more interested and responsive to the topic. The *intelligibility* of the speaker's voice, the extent to which the spoken message is heard and understood, is defined by aspects such as appropriate vocal rate, volume, articulation, correct use of pronunciation and grammar, and limited use of fillers (e.g., "uh," "um," "like," "ok," etc.) and pauses. *Vocal variation*, such as altering pitch, rate, or volume, and pausing at appropriate points in the speech can add emphasis to a particular word or thought and assists in avoiding a monotonous, boring delivery.

Physical or nonverbal aspects of the speaker such as appearance, eye contact, facial expressions, and gestures are equally important to a successful presentation. Attire and grooming should be appropriate for the audience or may create distraction or loss of speaker credibility. While tasteful "student apparel" may be suitable for speaking in front of classmates, professional wear is proper for more formal presentations. Direct eye contact with audience members is likely the most important of the physical characteristics of speech delivery. As in interpersonal communication, looking at the individual members of the audience while speaking helps to maintain attention and create connections with the listeners. Varying facial expressions and gestures with the head, arms, and hands can add emphasis or further define the spoken message, in addition to enlivening what would otherwise be a statue-like presenter.

> Surveys show that the top fear reported by Americans— even greater than the fear of dying—is public speaking (Bovee, 2001).

Self-confidence and maintaining poise through the delivery are key qualities for an effective speaker and are most influenced by anxiety issues. Almost everyone, including the most experienced speaker, is likely to feel some form of nervousness before speaking publicly. It is reassuring to know that you are not alone in feeling this type of discomfort. Understanding the cause and knowing the symptoms of public speaking anxiety can help you deal with it in a positive way.

Fears of inadequacy (in physical appearance or knowledge), of stating incorrect information, of criticism by the audience, or of something "going wrong" during the presentation are typical causes of apprehension when speaking in front of others. A variety of physical symptoms may be experienced by the speaker who is apprehensive, some of which may or may not be apparent to listeners: accelerated heart beat, queasiness, stomach "butterflies," sweating, flushing of the face, dryness of the mouth, heavy breathing, excessive swallowing or clearing of the throat; speech that is rapid, shaky, low in volume, or monotonous; disfluent speech such as stuttering, blocking, pausing inappropriately, or excessively using fillers; restricted head or body movement, lack of hand or arm gestures, pacing, wringing of hands, tapping of fingers; and lack of eye contact.

As speech anxiety will be a likely occurrence, it is useful to learn strategies to help control the effects.

Preparation

A common cause of speech apprehension is the fear of unanticipated situations that may arise during the presentation. Being prepared for the environment in which the speech is to take place and for possible mishaps during the delivery will help alleviate this concern. If possible, it is very helpful to view the room in which you are speaking beforehand in order to familiarize yourself with the physical aspects of the room setting such as size, lighting, the speaking location, and placement of audio-visual equipment. It is very unsettling to think that a technical problem may make a computer-generated presentation undeliverable after all the effort put into the preparation. Make sure you are familiar with the equipment to be used and that you can quickly summon technical assistance if a problem arises. Although it is unlikely, be prepared for the possibility of a complete equipment malfunction and the need to deliver the speech without audio-visual assistance. For this scenario, bring a complete copy of the slides from the computer-generated presentation as your reference. If isolated audio or video segments fail without resolution of the problem, you can summarize the content to the audience or have substitute material ready. Send your computer-generated presentation to yourself in an e-mail attachment, so that you have a back-up if your disk or flash drive is lost or malfunctions. Also, arrive early and install your presentation onto the desktop of the computer, as both access to and advancing/reversing your slides will be faster.

Practice

This is probably the most significant aspect of speech preparation in terms of strengthening and polishing the delivery. An added bonus is that practice leads to familiarity and comfort with the presentation, building confidence that can help to reduce stress. While there is no magic number as to how many times you should practice, do so until you have learned and can speak unassisted about the main components of the presentation. Ways to practice include speaking the presentation alone quietly or aloud, in front of a mirror or small audience of friends or family, or videotaping and then viewing yourself. Most importantly, be sure to practice on any equipment to be used so that you are sure of the operation and compatibility of any special effects that you plan to use.

Confidence

Don't underestimate the power of positive thinking. If you are prepared and have practiced your speech, you have every reason to believe you will deliver a good one. Also remember that if you do feel nervous, most often audience members will not notice, so relax.

Tips for Delivering the Speech

1. *Be confident and enthusiastic.* A positive attitude and energetic tone will *motivate the audience to listen*.
2. *Speak clearly.* Make sure you are not speaking rapidly and that your vocal volume is appropriate. If a microphone is used, check that it is working and not producing a booming or distorted sound.
3. *Dress and groom appropriately.* "Clinic dress" is a good rule of thumb. You want your audience to listen to you, not to be distracted by your outfit, hairstyle, or accessories.
4. *Establish eye contact with the audience.* This shows that you are confident and welcoming your audience to listen. Try to vary your eye contact among different listeners rather than focusing on the same few individuals.

5. *Use facial expressions and body gestures.* Avoid being stiff; being animated maintains the audience's attention and can add emphasis to your statements.
6. *Don't read the presentation or information projected onto slides.* You should be able to talk comfortably about the material in your presentation once prompted by a main or subpoint listed on index cards or on computer-projected slides. The spoken text is more casual and informal than written text. In oral presentation it is appropriate to use the first person pronouns *I*, *we*, and *you*, rather than *the speaker* and *the audience*. Spoken presentation is more redundant, and generally has shorter sentences than written text.

Sample Computer-Generated Presentation

Following is the introduction to an all-day symposium, delivered by the first author. The slide is followed by the oral text, which is roughly equivalent to the extemporaneous presentation. A reminder, in the form of XX, is used to indicate that it is necessary to move forward to the next slide. (Begin with Figure 6–1.)

Welcome to the symposium. Some preliminary announce-ments: XX (Figure 6–2).

1. Make sure you have Continuing Education forms if you want ASHA CEUs. Partial credit (0.3 CEUs) will be available for those attending only the morning or afternoon session.
2. Lunch break from 12:30 to 2:00. There is a restaurant list on the registration desk. Coffee and snacks are available on this level at 365 Express.
3. There is a display case of historical books on stuttering and original letters from Wendell Johnson and others in the registration area, thanks to Prof. Emeritus Robert Rieber.
4. Rest rooms are located in the back of the hall.
5. There are microphones on stands on both sides of the room. We will invite you to ask questions after each presentation, as time permits. XX (Figure 6–3).

Symposium on Ethics and The Tudor Study: Implications for Research in Stuttering

Friday, December 13, 2002

Baisley Powell Elebash Recital Hall

The Graduate Center, CUNY

Figure 6–1. Sample PowerPoint slide 1.

Announcements

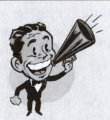

- ASHA CEUS (0.3)

- lunch break from 12:30–2:00

- display case on stuttering in registration area

- rest rooms located in the back of the hall

- questions welcome !!

Figure 6–2. Sample PowerPoint slide 2.

SPONSORS

- Ph.D. Program in Speech and Hearing Sciences, The Graduate Center, CUNY
- Continuing Education and Public Programs, The Graduate Center, CUNY
- The Malcolm Fraser Foundation
- Lehman College, CUNY (for CEUs)

Figure 6–3. Sample PowerPoint slide 3.

We are grateful to our sponsors for supporting this symposium. Please let me know at the break if you would like more information about our PhD program.

It is tempting and dangerous in a conference dealing with ethics to seize the moral high ground. XX (Figure 6-4)

Cicero warns us about the dangers of hubris. It is probably better if we think of this symposium more as an academic exercise than as a forum to respond to all the ethical issues posed by the Tudor study. That said, we will be looking in detail at Wendell Johnson's diagnosogenic or semantogenic theory, which most of us learned in our undergraduate study.

The theoretical physicist Stephen Hawking, who as you may know suffers from ALS and severe dysarthria, proposed a definition of a good theory. XX (Figure 6-5)

If the predictions agree with the observations, the theory survives that test, though it can never be proven to be correct. On the other hand, if the observations disagree with the predictions, we have to discard or modify the theory. XX (Figure 6-6)

"Why, upon the very books in which they bid us scorn ambition philosophers inscribe their names."

--Cicero

Figure 6–4. Sample PowerPoint slide 4.

Stephen Hawking's definition of a good theory

- Describe a large range of phenomena on the basis of a few simple postulates.
- Make definite predictions that can be tested.

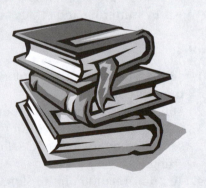

Figure 6–5. Sample PowerPoint slide 5.

> "(At least, that is what is supposed to happen. In practice, people often question the accuracy of the observations and the reliability and moral character of those making the observations.)"
>
> Hawking, S. *The universe in a nutshell*. New York: Bantam, p. 31

Figure 6–6. Sample PowerPoint slide 6.

If we think of theories as somewhat sacred, the reality of those charged with testing them is rather more profane.

We are about to begin a critical review not only of the Tudor study, which is, after all, no more or less than a 63-year-old master's thesis, but also a critical look at the issues of diagnosis in stuttering and ethics in scientific research.

Notes:

1. Simple slide design and color scheme, uniform throughout the presentation.
2. Minimal use of images to complement the slide text
3. Use of short phrases with few lines of text per slide; thoughts separated by use of bullets, line spacing, or contrasted font sizing.
4. Text information on the slide was referred to, but not read verbatim in the oral presentation.

References

Bovee, C. L. (2001). *Contemporary public speaking* (2nd ed.). San Diego, CA: Collegiate Press.

Grice, G. L., & Skinner, J. F. (1998). *Mastering public speaking* (3rd ed.). Needham Heights, MA: Allyn and Bacon.

Miculka, J. (1999). *Speaking for success*. Cincinnati, OH: South-Western Educational Publishing.

O'Hair, D., Friedrich, G. W., Wiemann, J. M., & Wiemann, M. O. (1997). *Competent communication* (2nd ed.). New York: St. Martin's Press.

Seiler, W. J., & Beall, M. L. (1999). *Communication: Making connections* (4th ed.). Boston: Allyn and Bacon.

Treholm, S. (1999). *Thinking through communication: An introduction to the study of human communication* (2nd ed.). Needham Heights, MA: Allyn and Bacon.

Zarefsky, D. (2002). *Public speaking: Strategies for success* (3rd ed.). Boston: Allyn and Bacon.

Zayas-Baya, E. P. (1977). Instructional media in the total language picture. *International Journal of Instructional Media*, 145–150.

EXERCISES

1. Which of the following is *not* one of the four methods of delivery of oral presentations?

   a. impromptu
   b. choral
   c. memorized
   d. manuscript
   e. extemporaneous

2. The research involved in oral presentation:

   a. is the same for all types of speeches
   b. does not require a reference list
   c. has looser rules for ethics and plagiarism
   d. should follow the same guidelines used in the writing of a research paper
   e. should not contain too many facts, which may be boring to the listener

3. In developing a speech:

   a. prepare the introduction, body, and conclusion in that order, since that is the order of presentation of the speech
   b. identify the *main points*, or major subdivisions, and organize them in a logical sequence for the introduction
   c. prepare forms of support by providing examples, references, or statistics, presented visually by tables, figures, or other images or in audio-video format
   d. always start with humor in the form of a short story or joke, since a main purpose of the introduction is to gain the attention of the audience
   e. conclude by saying, "The end" or "That's it," so the audience knows you are finished

4. In outlining the presentation:

   a. use sentence fragments in preparing and delivering the speech
   b. supporting a main point requires that there be at least two subpoints

    c. create a *speaker's outline*, using complete sentences

    d. use a Harvard outline, alternating Roman numerals and Arabic numbers

    e. use only main points and subpoints, because more detail will be too hard to follow

5. In delivering the oral presentation:

    a. always use computer-generated stimuli

    b. read the information on the PowerPoint (or other software program) slide

    c. keep the number of words per slide at 100 or fewer

    d. use as many "bells and whistles" in the form of animation and sound effects as possible, to maintain the audience's attention

    e. refer to the information on the slide, but never read it to your audience

ANSWERS

1. The answer is *b*. In impromptu or spontaneous speeches, oral presentations do not require some level of preparation in a written form of the speech and in practice of the delivery. A memorized delivery is one where the speech has been committed to memory from a prepared script. The manuscript delivery is one that is read word for word. The extemporaneous method, the most common form used in classrooms and general public speaking, is a combination of the three styles where notes or an outline is used with a high level of spontaneity in the delivery.

2. The answer is *d*. Statements made by the speaker should be supported by facts either stated in the presentation or in a printed reference list. Orally presented information is bound by the same principles of ethics and plagiarism as the written form.

3. The answer is *c*. Prepare the speech in any order, but the order of presentation is always introduction, body, and conclusion. The *main points*, or major subdivisions, belong in the body of the speech. Humor does not work on every occasion, and a strategy must be chosen carefully so that it is appropriate to the nature of the topic, composition of the audience, and comfort level of the speaker. Finally, the goal of the conclusion is to end the talk by concisely summarizing the main points as reinforcement of the message and providing final thoughts or suggestions.

4. The answer is *b*. This style is based on the idea that breaking something results in at least two pieces. Use complete sentences in preparing the speech, but key words or phrases in creating the speaker's outline used to deliver the speech. The Harvard outline uses uppercase Roman numerals, followed by indented capital letters, Arabic numbers, lowercase letters, and lowercase Roman numerals. Use of main points, subpoints, and supporting points depends on the sophistication level of the audience.

5. The answer is *e*. Computer-generated presentation is optional in a speech, and should be used according to the rules in this chapter . There are few experiences more boring than sitting through a speech where the slides are read aloud verbatim. Try for a limit of 25 words on a single slide; use bulleted sentences or phrases to separate thoughts. Use pictures, cartoons, jokes, racing car noises, and other "enhancements" sparingly, so that their effect will be magnified when you do use them.

CHAPTER 7

The Diagnostic Report

The diagnostic report represents a comprehensive written account of the clinical assessment/evaluation and serves two general purposes. First, the report is a professional document (and thus a legal document; see discussion below) and written evidence of the clinical service. Second, the diagnostic report is often sent to other professionals involved with the case, as the source of or for referral. As such diagnostic reports, though they may differ among clinics, are generally written in formal, professional language. We begin this chapter with rules for diagnosis and end with strategies for writing the diagnostic report, with guidelines specific to speech-language pathology or audiology.

Diagnostic Labeling

A recent article in *The New York Times* (Carey, 2007) reported a 40-fold increase in the number of American children and adolescents who were treated for bipolar disorder in the decade from 1994 to 2003. Almost certainly, the number has increased further since then. There is little concern about the likelihood of a vast increase in incidence of bipolar disorder, as the consensus is that doctors currently use the diagnosis more aggressively than before. The startling magnitude of the increase in diagnosis intensifies the debate over the validity and reliability of the diagnosis. If the term *bipolar disorder* is applied as a catchall for any child exhibiting explosive or aggressive behaviors, then far too many children are being treated with powerful psychoactive drugs with few demonstrable benefits and many potentially serious side effects.

The field of communication sciences and disorders is hardly exempt from faddish behavior in applying diagnostic labels. The term *cluttering* was widely used in the 1960s and 1970s to describe rapid-fire, indistinct speech with some word-finding difficulty and lack of awareness of difficulty by the speaker. This may be seen as a result of adopting the theories of Deso Weiss (1964), but the term subsequently fell into disuse. It may be reviving currently, in part because of new research efforts (see, for example, St. Louis & Myers, 2007).

Similarly, the term *central auditory processing disorder* (CAPD) has frequently been misused to label individuals, particularly children, who present with listening problems in the absence of apparent hearing loss. Though true CAPD is a deficit of the auditory modality, comparable listening difficulties may be noted in children with attention deficit hyperactivity disorder (ADHD), language impairment, or learning disability, rendering a possible misdiagnosis of CAPD. Following decades of inconsistency on the definition, assessment, and remediation of CAPD, ASHA organized a Task Force on Central Auditory Processing in 1993, which arrived at consensus on the issues (ASHA, 1996; 2005).

Threats to Accurate Diagnosis

Problems in written diagnostic reports may be traced to the following two threats:

- *Polytypicality:* Schwartz (1984) noted shortcomings in the descriptors for aphasia. She noted that adults with aphasia commonly display language characteristics that cross diagnostic boundaries. That is, they are polytypic in nature. It is not unusual for a patient with Broca's aphasia, for example, to have difficulty in auditory comprehension, an impairment listed among the principal diagnostic characteristics of Wernicke's aphasia. As noted in Diagnostic Rule 1 below, it is appropriate to write about the speech, language, and hearing characteristics of the individual, rather than merely assigning a label, especially if the diagnostic category is not obvious.
- *Dumping it in the chocolate:* One of the authors (RG) supported himself through college by working in an ice cream

factory. As an interesting aside, he had firsthand experience with homeostasis, or the body's tendency to maintain itself in an essentially healthy state. Alternating half-hour shifts in the ice box, where the temperature was −42°, with half-hour shifts outside, where the temperature was as high as 90° in the summer, his internal temperature stayed at 98.6°. Occasionally, at the end of the workday there was excess ice cream mix. The next day's run would start with chocolate, and the excess mix would be blended in. Chocolate was strong enough in flavor and color to absorb the leftover.

There are frequent instances in our professions where we metaphorically dump the diagnosis in the chocolate. Some gratuitous examples occur in the diagnosis of "quirky" children. Catch-all terms begin at birth, where the diagnosis of FLK (for *funny-looking kid*; see Chapter 1) has only recently been discontinued. Children whose language impairment is presented in the absence of other disorders are classified as having *specific language impairment* (SLI). Not so many years ago, *aphasia in children* was the preferred classification. In the Middle Ages, the medical diagnosis for quirky children was *humors of the liver*; more recently, the children were diagnosed with brain fever, minimum brain damage, and minimal cerebral dysfunction. Currently, the chocolate into which these children's problems are dumped is the reticulo-limbic complex.

Rules for Diagnosis

Rule 1

Say what the client does, not what the client is. In other words, report behaviors and limit the number of diagnostic labels.

Nobody likes to read an overlong diagnostic report. Efforts at brevity are laudable, and a particular strategy for summarizing case history information appears later in this chapter. However, a haphazard use of diagnostic labels often does more harm than good. A general application of Rule 1 is to follow any diagnostic label with the phrase, *characterized by* . . . Although this rule may seem similar to the signing statements of a U.S. President, indicating the applications and limitations of a new law (which may or may not be constitutional), the rule addresses the need of school districts and third-party payers for a diagnostic label, and summarizes the areas of deficit to be addressed in therapy.

A diagnostic report is a legal document. In the following trial transcriptions, the first author was employed by the defense as an expert witness, to counteract claims put forth by the plaintiff that were supported by a speech-language pathologist. Although trial transcriptions are a matter of public record, names and identifying information were changed here. Certifying a witness as an expert allows that individual to offer opinions; a witness who is not certified as an expert can offer only facts. Certification as an expert may be based on academic standing (a rank of full professor, not adjunct instructor), publications (which have been peer-reviewed), or experience (many years in positions of high responsibility).

The judge is indicated as *the court*; the first author is *the witness*.

> *The Court:* In your opinion, using these two documents [Exhibit H and Exhibit RR], has Ms. B been misdiagnosed?

> *The Witness:* Yes. Let me give two examples in the speech-language evaluation report where Ms. B was misdiagnosed.

> The first diagnostic term that was used in error was *paragrammatism*. That is on page 2. Here we have, "Paragrammatisms and superfluous words were noted in writing and speech." We have as an example that sentence beginning, "Lee Atwater was a tumor."

> The definition of paragrammatism is that it occurs in Wernicke's aphasia, and that it is characterized by substitutions of functors. A functor is what might be called a helping word as opposed to a substantive or a lexical word. So under functors we look at things like prepositions, articles, conjunctions, auxiliary verbs. And what I am interpreting here is that the justification for the diagnosis of paragrammatism is the word "was" after "Lee Atwater" when the word should have been "had." "Lee Atwater had a tumor," as opposed to, "Lee Atwater was a tumor."

The problem is that paragrammatism, as I said, occurs in posterior aphasia. There was no evidence and no claim in this diagnostic report that the patient had any kind of posterior aphasia. To the contrary, there is significant evidence that the aphasia was an anterior type, that is, the kind of aphasia that is characterized by halting, effortful speech, by problems with articulation. For example, the apraxias that are referred to do not accompany posterior aphasias or Wernicke's aphasia. These apraxias accompany anterior or Broca's aphasia, as it was referred to here.

So the problem that I see with paragrammatism is that it doesn't belong as a diagnostic classification with this kind of patient.

Furthermore, the one example here, the word "was" which follows "Lee Atwater," was an example of a functor substitution. However, if we can look for a moment at Exhibit RR—I am going to try and find it; this is another large document here—we have an example where a paragrammatism was described— if I don't find it, let me explain it to you—where a paragrammatism was described, and the example given was the substitution of a substantive word rather than a functor word.

What I am saying is that a paragrammatism has to be a grammatical or a syntactic error. The example which had something to do with the organization of the government in the City of New York, I believe it was on 6/8—I am just not getting it here—the example was one of a semantic error rather than a syntactic error.

So the term "paragrammatism" was used incorrectly and was also used to describe a symptom that would occur in a different kind of aphasia.

The other misdiagnosis has to do with, again, going back to Exhibit H, the bottom of page 2: "Impression. Presenting persistent aphasia is Broca and conduction in type." Let me speak to that.

This cannot be. The aphasia cannot be Broca and conduction in type. Broca's aphasia is nonfluent aphasia. Conduction aphasia is fluent aphasia. A person can't be fluent and nonfluent at the same time.

Conduction aphasia is characterized by, among other things, a disproportionately large number of errors in repetition, as opposed to other language modalities tested.

Now, the references to repetition, again in Exhibit H, top of the page, page 2, "Repetition (sentences) was impaired and variable." Going back, bottom of the page under "Impression," we have "manifested and mildly impaired repetition."

Repetition, according to these notes, even if it was mildly impaired, was not impaired in a disproportionately significant way to other modalities tested.

Furthermore, in Exhibit RR, the first page, dated 5/14, we have a note: "Repetition intact."

The last thing I want to say about conduction aphasia is that classically Broca's area, if Ms. A was following the model of the localizationist, Broca's area is classically associated with the third frontal convolution on the left side of the brain, and Broca's aphasia then would presumably follow a lesion in that area. Conduction aphasia would presumably follow a lesion in the arcuate fasciculus, which is the neural pathway connecting Wernicke's area to Broca's area. There was no evidence and no claim that there was any damage to the arcuate fasciculus.

What I am troubled by is the tendency to form diagnostic categories or label diagnostic categories based on skimpy evidence and done in an illogical manner.

As a final note to Rule 1, all of the above criticisms might have been avoided if the speech-language pathologist, Ms. A, had described the characteristics of Ms. B's language disorder, rather than the labels that she used in error. There is no shame in using the term *nonfluent aphasia* if you are not sure of such terms as Broca's aphasia, *conduction aphasia*, or *paragrammatism*. In fact, describing aphasia as nonfluent is probably more useful, because it describes an aspect of the communication disorder that needs to be addressed in therapy.

Rule 2

Be an educated consumer of tests and measures. Although the doctorate is generally seen as the degree associated with the production of research, all audiologists and speech-language pathologists must understand research methodology.

The authors recall discussions with the late Ira Ventry, when he was developing ideas for a book on research methods in communication sciences and disorders. The current edition of the book (Schiavetti & Metz, 2006) provides the basis for the information that follows.

Reliability means precision of measurement. It is assessed by examining the consistency or stability of a test or measure. *Validity* means generalizability of the data. It means the degree to which a test measures what it purports to measure. It means truth or correctness or reality of measurement. A butcher's scale may consistently and precisely weigh meat at ½ pound over the true or correct weight. It is reliable, but not valid. On the other hand, it is not possible for a test to be valid without being reliable.

There are three ways to check reliability of a test or measurement.

1. *Test-retest reliability:* Completely repeat the test. If the test is repeated with the same client after a latency period (to avoid the practice effect or learning to learn), but within a reasonable period of time (to avoid effects of maturation or spontaneous recovery), the score should be pretty much the same as it was in the first administration of the test.
2. *Parallel or equivalent form:* Examine consistency of the results across the two equivalent forms. These forms are used when testing two different modalities or two different conditions (see, for example, time-altered word association tests by Goldfarb & Halpern, 1981).

3. *Split-half:* Subdivide the test or measure into two equivalent parts (usually odd-even) to examine consistency of these parts. This is similar to parallel or equivalent forms, where one half may be used at the beginning of therapy as a baseline measure, and the other half at the end of therapy for baseline recovery.

Another type of reliability, called inter-rater or inter-scorer reliability, is used in experimental research, to ensure that there are no significant differences in scores assigned, and is based only on how people score the data.

There are also three ways to establish the validity of a test or measure.

1. *Content validity:* Logically or rationally evaluate items on a test to see how well they reflect what the tester wishes to measure, using subjective procedures.
2. *Criterion validity:* See how well the test or measure correlates with some outside validating criterion. There are two types of criterion validity.
   a. *Concurrent validity:* Administer a test or measure and an outside validating criterion at the same time. For example, the first edition of the *Peabody Picture Vocabulary Test* used an IQ test as a measure of concurrent validity, and indicated an equivalent IQ score based solely on this test of receptive vocabulary (It no longer has a space to report an IQ score.). A key concept is that an *outside* validating criterion is used. Hildred Schuell (1966; 1973) assessed concurrent validity using two versions of the same test (the short and long forms of the *Minnesota Test for Differential Diagnosis of Aphasia* [MTDDA]), a questionable strategy also used to compare the third and fourth editions of the *Clinical Evaluation of Language Functioning*. However, Schuell determined that the short form of the MTDDA was not valid.
   b. *Predictive validity:* Use a test or measure to predict some future behavior. Administer the test, allow time to elapse, and then administer the criterion measure. For example, use the *Boston Naming Test* (BNT) as a baseline measure and the *Porch Index of Communicative Ability* (PICA) to predict how much an adult might be expected to improve

word retrieval following therapy for aphasia, and then give the BNT at the final therapy session. See how the differences in the BNT correspond to the "HOAP slope" predicted on the PICA. Note that IQ tests, such as the *Stanford-Binet* or the *Wechsler Intelligence Scale for Children*, are predictive tests. An IQ score is properly used to predict how well a child may be expected to perform in school.

3. *Construct validity:* Assess the degree to which a test or measure reflects some theory or explanation of the characteristic to be measured. The test or measure should confirm the theory if the test is valid *and* if the theory is correct. For example, a theory might predict that post-stroke and typical adults might use vocabulary differently. If the test or measure confirmed this, then the measure would have construct validity with respect to that aspect of the theory. However, if the theory has been discredited, as has Osgood's notion that language is based on the sum of a set of specific abilities, then no manner of validity in the content of the *Illinois Test of Psycholinguistic Ability* (short of attempting to confirm another theory) will yield construct validity.

Rule 3

Beware of "clinicese." Clients may exhibit behaviors in the clinic that they do not generalize outside of the speech and hearing center.

Young children, particularly those with disfluencies, may present dramatically different patterns of communication disorders, depending on context. For example, a child may stutter more when evaluated by "Dr. Goldfarb," who is wearing a tie and a lab coat, than when "Bob" conducts the same evaluation wearing casual clothing.

Yaruss, LaSalle, and Conture (1998) recommended a three-part evaluation to determine quantitative and qualitative differences in arriving at a diagnosis of stuttering:

1. conversational interaction between child and caregiver(s) (20 to 30 minutes);
2. evaluation of the child's speech, language, and related behaviors (60 to 90 minutes); and
3. an interview of the child's caregiver(s) (45 to 60 minutes).

This 3-hour procedure may be unrealistic in many work settings. However, the traditional method of assessing a wide variety of interacting psychosocial, psycholinguistic, and physiologic variables will likely take longer and may not differentiate among children at risk for stuttering.

Yaruss et al. (1998) used measures of speech fluency, measures of speech and language development, and other measures, including the child's diadochokinetic rate and parents' speaking rates to determine presence of a pathological condition. There was still considerable overlap between children recommended for reevaluation and those who received neither treatment nor reevaluation. "It would seem essentially impossible to develop absolute criteria for determining which children should receive which diagnostic recommendation" (Yaruss et al, 1998, p.72).

Rule 4

Do differential diagnosis when appropriate. Diagnostically related groups (sometimes abbreviated as DRGs) often present similar audiometric and/or language profiles.

Our research has proceeded from the premise that linguistic data can aid in the differential diagnosis of diagnostically related groups. The following case study (Goldfarb, 2006b) illustrates the need for differential diagnosis, and assumes the reader to be a physician, nurse, or social worker at University Hospital:

> An elderly homeless man, identified as Mr. X because he cannot say his name, has been admitted with what the emergency room physician described as "disorganized language." The patient has no identification, no documented medical history, and has not yet had brain imaging studies. You have been asked to determine if the disorganized language represents fluent aphasia, the language of schizophrenia, or the language of dementia.

The patient is referred to a speech-language pathologist at University Hospital. Evaluation of Mr. X's language reveals preservation of prosody, phonology, morphology, and syntax, with disturbances in semantics and pragmatics. This still fits the pattern of the diagnostically related groups of fluent aphasia, the language of Alzheimer and multi-infarct dementia, and the language of chronic undifferentiated schizophrenia.

In a standard diagnostic audiologic evaluation, several subtests within the complete battery of testing provide information on a patient's middle ear and hearing status (degree, configuration, and type of hearing loss). However, several auditory or vestibular pathologies may exhibit similar audiometric profiles, warranting further differential diagnosis before an appropriate treatment plan can be implemented. Characteristics such as a report of sudden hearing loss and dizziness along with audiometric findings of unilateral sensorineural hearing loss and normal middle ear function may be associated with disorders such as Ménière's disease, acoustic neuritis, or acoustic tumor. In this case, the audiologist may need to perform further diagnostic tests such as auditory brainstem response testing (ABR) or electronystagmography (ENG) in order to assist the physician in a medical diagnosis.

Rule 5

Obey the limits of our scope of practice. Provide diagnostic labels that relate to the communicative disorder, not the medical cause.

It is no wonder patients frequently assume audiologists are physicians; given recent changes in ASHA certification standards (Council For Clinical Certification in Audiology and Speech-Language Pathology of the American Speech-Language-Hearing Association, 2007) most now hold the "doctor" title, typically work in a medical setting, and perform many "medical-like" tasks such as otoscopy, ABR, ENG, and cerumen removal. It is also logical that the audiologist, who upon otoscopic examination detects fluid bubbles and redness of the tympanic membrane and finds conductive hearing loss following audiometric testing with reduced tympanometric peak admittance, will conclude *otitis media* as the underlying cause of pathology. Nonetheless, however obvious the disorder, it is not within the audiologist's scope of practice to provide a medical label. Similarly, the speech-language pathologist who evaluates an adult with imprecise articulation, word-finding deficits, and right facial droop may diagnose aphasia and dysarthria, but not the underlying stroke. The role of the communicative disorders specialist, audiologist or speech-language pathologist, is to describe and identify the disorder and to refer the patient for medical diagnosis of the cause (in these examples, middle ear pathology and brain damage).

Writing the Diagnostic Report

A generation ago, Dr. Aaron Smith tended to highlight his presentations to the Academy of Aphasia by noting that, "The patient doesn't lie." The current television incarnation of Sherlock Holmes, Dr. Gregory House, tends to tell his Dr. Watson (Dr. Wilson on TV) that the patient always lies. In Dr. House's case the resolution between the received wisdom and the awful truth involves a heavy dose of misogyny as well as breaking and entering, and takes 1 hour. In Dr. Smith's case, the differences between the patient's language behavior and the population norms described in professional literature are not resolved.

The large-sample studies reported in our journals are essential to provide the theoretical bases for our professions and to permit generalization of the findings to untested populations. However, there are two problems in using clinical data to support or disconfirm hypotheses. The first is that language, speech, and hearing are incredibly complex processes. The underlying basis for the disorder is often debatable, especially in speech-language pathology (see Goldfarb, 2006a, for a description of the atheoretical discipline of stuttering). Our tendency toward reductionism in thinking and writing works better in audiology, which is a more mature science, but is still a reflection of what we may call *physics envy*. Boiling down cascades of data into a more manageable size is typical of the natural sciences, but does not work very well in the behavioral sciences. The second problem is that clinical data reflect the client's, not the population's, language, speech, and hearing. As we have learned in Diagnostic Labeling above, the client's communication disorder may cross typical categorical boundaries, and may be uniquely the individual's own, in terms of type and severity of disorder. That is why we always put the individual first in our descriptions; an individual who stutters, rather than a stutterer. It is also why we must be logical in our report writing.

The Logic of Report Writing

If only fools are kind, Alfie,
Then I guess it's wise to be cruel.

Although Burt Bacharach is to be commended for the excellence of his song writing, his logic is flawed. Beginning with the thesis of "if p, then q," there are four constructions, only two of which are logical. Accordingly,

Statement: if p then q

Converse: if q then p

Inverse: if not p then not q

Contrapositive: if not q then not p

In the *Alfie* song, the logical thesis, which is accepted here for argument's sake, is, *If a person is kind (p), then that person is a fool (q).* The actual lines of the song represent the inverse of the argument, which is not logical. Examples from our discipline follow.

Thesis: If there is a lesion in Broca's area (p), then there will be a word retrieval deficit (q). This statement is accepted as logical.

Inverse: If there is not a lesion in Broca's area, then there will not be a word retrieval deficit. This statement is not logical.

Converse: If there is a word retrieval deficit, then there will be a lesion in Broca's area. This statement is not logical.

Contrapositive: If there is not a word retrieval deficit, then there will not be a lesion in Broca's area. This statement is logical.

Curiously, the patient Broca described in 1861 (called "Tan" or "Tant" because that was his stereotypic utterance) probably did not have Broca's aphasia. Broca described Tant as having *aphémie*, or aphemia, which corresponds to apraxia of speech, rather than having *aphasie*, the French word which corresponds to aphasia. In addition, Tant's lesion was in the anterior portion of the third frontal convolution in the left hemisphere, rather than the posterior portion described as Broca's area. Damasio (2008) reviewed the case of Tant and concluded that he must have suffered from global aphasia. So Broca's patient didn't have Broca's aphasia, nor did he have a lesion in Broca's area.

The Diagnostic Report Format

Though the specific format and subheadings of the diagnostic report may differ among clinics, most follow a commonly used medical organizational outline known as *SOAP* (S = *subjective*; O = *objective*; A = *assessment*; P = *plan*).

The subjective section (a.k.a. referral, background information, or history) includes the client's biographical information, reason for referral, and relevant developmental (with a pediatric client), medical, and communicative history. The objective part (a.k.a. assessment information; *note*: this term differs from the SOAP definition of assessment; see below) incorporates all the information obtained during the session, including observed behaviors and elicited test procedures and outcomes. The information obtained from the subjective and objective sections is synthesized to formulate a diagnostic statement, often headed in a section entitled, "Clinical Impressions" (in the SOAP format this section is referred to as assessment). Finally, a plan (a.k.a. recommendations) for treatment, further recommendations, and follow-up is indicated.

Guidelines for Writing Diagnostic Reports in Speech-Language Pathology and Audiology

Writing Aspects

1. Always write in complete, grammatically correct sentences. Use professional books, not a dictionary, to make sure you are using the appropriate terminology and that terms are spelled correctly.
2. Write clearly and present the information accurately.

3. Be concise; state only the relevant information of the case. Reports that are too lengthy will typically not be read thoroughly.

Format

Follow the diagnostic report format of the institution. Although the format may vary according to site, the following specifics are usually considered:

1. Include all section headings (using boldface, underline, and italics as indicated by the institution; see headings below).
2. Adhere to the format regarding positioning, lettering, and underlining of the section headings (e.g., some may be centered, some flush with the left margin; the report title is usually all capitals; section headings may be underlined).
3. Include the names of students (designated as *clinical interns*), as well as the name and credentials of the clinical supervisor.

Sections of the Diagnostic Report

Referral Information[1]

Include full name of client, age, gender, name of treatment center, referral source, name of person accompanying client to evaluation, name of informant, reliability of informant to provide background information, reason for referral, and statement of problem.

Background Information[1]

Document case history information pertinent to the disorder and appropriate to the client.

For a child:

1. Child's prenatal and birth history, including maternal health; medications during pregnancy, labor, and delivery; length of pregnancy, indicating pre- or post-term; type of delivery

---

[1]In some report formats, as is typical in audiology, *Referral* and *Background Information* may be combined into a *History* section.

(using *C-section* as an abbreviation for caesarian section, but not *SVD* as an abbreviation for spontaneous vaginal delivery); complications; neonatal health.

2. Child's developmental history for motor and speech-language development, indicating if ages of developmental milestones are within normal limits.

For a child or an adult:

1. Child's or adult's medical history, such as pertinent illnesses or injuries, hospitalizations, respiratory infections, allergies, ear infections and how treated, and medications.
2. Other pertinent evaluations and therapies, such as speech-language, audiological, psychological, and neurological.
3. Family, social, educational, and occupational history, indicating with whom client resides, primary language spoken if not English, peer relationships, and history of speech, language, hearing, and learning problems in family.

Assessment Information

Include information obtained during the diagnostic session, both observed and measured.

1. Report formal test scores in a table format.
2. Use narrative sections to *describe behaviors*, not to reiterate test scores (see above).

Clinical Impressions

Formulate a diagnostic statement of the problem. Provide a summary of relevant findings from the previous sections of the report, highlighting problem areas, etiology, and prognosis.

1. Do not report new information in this section.
2. Use behaviors and test scores previously reported as evidence to substantiate a diagnosis.

Recommendations

Recommendations may include a plan of treatment, further testing (continuation or follow-up), additional evaluations, and referral to other specialists. List the appropriate recommendations in order of importance. For example, if a medical referral is warranted, that should be indicated first.

Report Drafts

1. *Double-space report drafts* to facilitate editing and correcting by the supervisor.
2. *Maintain client anonymity*. Identify the client only by initials in drafts of reports, whether in e-mail, diskette, compact disc, or hard copy form. Remember that all these versions contain privileged and confidential information.
3. *Place final drafts of reports*, with the supervisor's signature, in the appropriate tray on the office administrator's desk. Sign in all reports in the log book.

Writing the History

In "Notes for Contributors" for the journal *Aphasiology*, submissions including reports of research with human participants should include the descriptive data identified by Brookshire (1983). These data include the following:

Age	Severity	Time since onset	Natural speaker
Type	Hearing	Education	Lateralization of damage
Sex	Vision	Etiology	
IQ	Hemianopia	Handedness	Localization of damage
Mood	Hemiparesis	Participant source	

These descriptors may not all be relevant to individuals who do not have brain damage, or to children, and the list should be expanded when writing a diagnostic report for an individual with hearing loss.

With so much information recommended, the first part of the diagnostic report can go on for several pages, so it is important to be concise. For example, consider the following summary:

> This 67-year-old, right-handed, English-speaking former
> construction worker with 12 years of education
> presented with a history of L CVA (3 mo. post-onset)

with resultant R hemiparesis and R homonymous hemianopia. He appeared alert and oriented × 3, wore corrective lenses and bilateral hearing aids, and appeared to be a reliable informant.

Some of the shorthand used, identified in Chapter 1, included *L* and *R* for *left* and *right*, *CVA* for *cerebrovascular accident*, *mo.* for *months*, and *oriented × 3* for *oriented to time, place, and person*. The two sentences (51 words) above provided 17 relevant pieces of case history information:

1. Age (67 years old)
2. Handedness (right-handed)
3. Natural speaker (English-speaking)
4. Previous employment (construction worker)
5. Education (12 years)
6. Medical diagnosis (CVA)
7. Localization of damage (L hemisphere)
8. Time since onset (3 mo.)
9. Lateralization of damage (R side of body)
10. Hemiparesis (present)
11. Hemianopia (present)
12. Sex (male, indicated by "he" to begin the second sentence)
13. Mood (alert)
14. Orientation (oriented to time, place, and person)
15. Vision (corrective lenses)
16. Hearing (bilaterally aided)
17. Reliability of information (reliable informant)

Diagnostic Report Format—Speech and Language

Name	Date of Evaluation
Address	Date of Birth
Address (2nd line)	Age (years:months for age <18)

Telephone Number
(Specify home, work, or cell, and include area codes.)

E-mail

Referral Information

Include full name of client, age, gender, name of treatment center, referral source, name of person accompanying client to evaluation, name of informant, reliability of informant to provide background information, reason for referral, and statement of problem.

Background Information

Document information pertinent to the disorder and appropriate to the client.

For a child:

1. Child's prenatal and birth history, including maternal health; medications during pregnancy, labor, and delivery; length of pregnancy, indicating pre- or post-term; type of delivery (using *C-section* as an abbreviation for caesarian section, but not *SVD* as an abbreviation for spontaneous vaginal delivery); complications; neonatal health.
2. Child's developmental history for motor and speech-language development, indicating if ages of developmental milestones are within normal limits.

For a child or an adult:

1. Child's or adult's medical history, such as pertinent illnesses or injuries, hospitalizations, respiratory infections, allergies, ear infections and how treated, and medications.
2. Other pertinent evaluations and therapies, such as speech-language, audiological, psychological, and neurological.
3. Family, social, educational, and occupational history, indicating with whom client resides, primary language spoken if not English, peer relationships, and history of speech, language, hearing, and learning problems in family.

Assessment Information

Write an introductory paragraph, citing behavioral observations, such as willingness to separate from the accompanying person;

cooperation and participation during assessment; attention span, eye-gaze, head and trunk orientation; activity level, remembering that *very active* is not the same as *hyperactive*; imitation of motor and speech behaviors, remembering that *echoic* is not the same as *echolalic*; and interaction behaviors.

Formal Testing (in table format)

Name of Test (use italics for test names)   *Results*

Raw Score

Age Equivalent

Percentile Rank

Standard Score

Pragmatics of Communication

Document form of communication, such as vocal, gestural, graphic; conversational skills, such as initiation, maintenance, elaboration, and termination of discourse topics; body posture and eye contact; turn-taking skills; requesting (action, information, clarification; comprehension/use of indirect requests involving modals, such as, *Would you close the door?*); contextual appropriateness of responses. Document level of demand for creativity, or communicative responsibility, when assessing disfluency.

Language Comprehension

Document responses to *yes-no*, *either-or*, and *wh-* questions; vocal and written directives (one-step and multistep, with simple and complex syntax); receptive vocabulary tasks, including sequential, confrontation, and associative naming; and reading comprehension tasks.

Language Production

Assess expressive vocabulary, and differentially diagnose word-retrieval impairment from vocabulary deficit; mean length of utterance as a word-morpheme index (the average of number of words plus number of morphemes per utterance, divided by 2, for at least 50 utterances); encoding of questions; syntax of constructions; narrative abilities; and written language skills.

Speech Production

Assess phonetic inventory, including sound substitutions, omissions, and distortions; phonemic inventory, including syllable shapes, and phonological processes used, with examples; overall intelligibility, comprehensibility, and stimulability.

Orofacial Examination and Feeding

If swallowing is not a primary concern, assess diadochokinesis in alternating and sequential motion rate tasks; facial symmetry, structure, and function; response to isometric and counter-resistance tasks for lips, tongue, cheeks, and mandible; tongue bulk and presence of fasciculations; velopharyngeal closure for speech and swallowing; self-feeding of liquids and solids.

If swallowing is a primary concern, assess frequency and percentage of swallowing characteristics on a clinical/bedside instrument such as the 28-item *Northwestern Dysphagia Patient Check Sheet*. Be prepared with liquid, puree, and solid bolus samples; be prepared to refer for videofluoroscopic swallowing evaluation.

Voice and Fluency

If voice and fluency are not primary concerns, report perceptual judgments of fluency, as well as vocal quality, resonance, pitch, and loudness.

If voice is a primary concern, in addition to the perceptual judgments above, report laboratory findings, such as fundamental frequency, maximum phonation time, s/z ratio, vital capacity, phonation quotient, and ability to shift from vegetative breathing to speech breathing. If fluency is a primary concern, in addition to the perceptual judgments above, report types, frequency, duration, and loci of disfluency; part-word and whole-word (or whole-phrase) repetitions; syllables stuttered divided by syllables spoken; secondary or associated behaviors; linguistic and situational behaviors affecting fluency; client's perceptions of fluency; and stimulability to modify fluency.

Cognition and Play

Include play only for young children. Assess parallel play, representative or symbolic play, and cooperative play; object permanence; means-to-an-end causality; conservation of continuous quantity; decentration from color to shape, size, and orientation; and problem-solving skills.

For older children and adults, assess cognitive tempo and cognitive style, and categorize as immediate-accurate, delayed-accurate, immediate-inaccurate, and delayed-inaccurate. Assess primacy (first stimulus) and recency (last stimulus) effects.

Audition

Report results of hearing screening or complete audiological evaluation, as well as response to sound at conversational levels.

Motor Skills

Include assessment of fine and gross motor skills, such as full-fist versus pincer grasp for young children, and writing with the non-dominant hand for adults with aphasia post-stroke.

Clinical Impressions

Justify your recommendations. Do not present new information in this section, but refer statements to prior assessment sections. Begin with full name of client and diagnosis (e.g., *Jane Doe, age 6:1, presents with a language production disorder, characterized by* . . .). Provide a summary of relevant findings, highlighting problem areas, etiology, and prognosis.

Recommendations

Indicate type (e.g., individual and group), frequency (e.g., three times per week for 9 weeks), and duration (e.g., 45-minute sessions) of therapy, as well as additional evaluations needed (e.g., audiological, psychological, educational). If you recommend speech-language therapy, end this paragraph with, *Initial goals of therapy should include . . .*

Clinical interns
(Names of students participating in evaluation)

Supervisor's name, degree, CCC-SLP

Speech-language pathologist

Institutional title (professor, clinical supervisor)

Diagnostic Protocol Worksheet—
Speech and Language

Client's Name   Date of Evaluation

Referral Information

Referral source

Informant

Informant reliability

Reason for concern

Background Information

For a Child

Prenatal and birth history

Speech-language developmental milestones

Motor development milestones

Medical history

For a Child or Adult

Other evaluations

Prior and current therapies

Client resides with

Primary language spoken at home

Family history of speech-language, hearing, learning problems

Educational and occupational information

Peer relationships

Favorite foods, TV shows, activities, best friend

Assessment Information

Behavioral observations

Is today's performance typical?

Pragmatics

Form of communication

Conversational skills

Eye contact and body orientation

Functional use of language

Communicative demand

Language Comprehension

Receptive vocabulary

Response to questions

   Yes-no

   Either-or

   Wh-

Ability to follow directions
  One-step commands
  Multiple-commission commands
Reading comprehension

Language Production

Expressive vocabulary

Encoding of questions

Content categories

Word-morpheme index for MLU

Morpho-syntactic skills

Word retrieval skills

Narrative abilities

Written language skills

Speech Production

Phonetic inventory

Sound substitutions, omissions, distortions

Phonemic inventory and syllable shapes

Phonological processes and examples

Speech intelligibility and comprehensibility

Stimulability

Orofacial Examination and Feeding

Facial symmetry

Structure of mandible, lips, teeth, tongue, palate, velum

Function of articulators

Diadochokinesis

Alternating motion rate

Sequential motion rate

Feeding for liquids, purees, solids

Drooling, dribbling

Voice

Quality

Resonance

Pitch (or *frequency*, if a laboratory measure)

Loudness (*volume* or *amplitude displacement*, if a laboratory measure)

Fluency

Blocks

Whole-word or phrase

Part-word

Repetitions

Prolongations

Associated/secondary mannerisms

Fluency ratio

Linguistic/environmental triggers

Cognition and Play

For a Child

Object permanence

Decentration

Conservation

Means/end

Play skills
   Parallel
   Representative/symbolic
   Cooperative

For an Adult

Imitation skills

Problem solving

Orientation to time, place, person, direction

Cognitive tempo/style

Audition

Testing results

Response to conversational levels

Motor Skills

Fine motor

Gross motor

Use of nondominant hand

Diagnostic Report Format—Audiology

See Martin and Clark, 2009; Northern, 1995; Stach, 1998.

Name	Date of Evaluation
Address	Date of Birth
Address (2nd line)	Age (years:months for age <18)

Telephone Number
(Specify home, work, or cell, and include area codes.)

E-mail

History

Include full name of the client, age, gender, referral source, name of person accompanying client to evaluation, name of informant (if not the client), reliability of informant to provide background information, reason for referral, and statement of problem. State whether this is a first or reevaluation. If this is a reevaluation, summarize the findings from the last session.

Document only information pertinent to the disorder and appropriate to the client.

1. For a child:
   a. Child's prenatal and birth history, including maternal health; medications during pregnancy, labor, and delivery; length of pregnancy, indicating pre- or post-term; type of delivery; complications; neonatal health.
   b. Child's developmental history for motor and speech-language development, indicating if ages of developmental milestones are within normal limits.
   c. Educational history including class grade, academic difficulties, special services.
   d. Behavioral issues such as hyperactivity, attention difficulty, etc.

2. For a child or an adult:
   a. Medical history, such as pertinent illnesses or injuries, hospitalizations, surgeries, respiratory infections, allergies, dizziness, medications, ear infections, ear pain, drainage.
   b. Hearing history, with description of current hearing status, hearing loss (if any) including onset, known cause, stability, and affected ear(s), amplification use, family history of hearing loss, tinnitus, noise exposure.
   c. Previous hearing tests and other pertinent evaluations and therapies, such as speech-language, psychological, and neurological.

Assessment Information

1. Write an introductory paragraph, citing only relevant behavioral observations, such as cooperation and participation during assessment; attention span, eye-gaze; reliability of testing.
2. If this is a reevaluation, compare findings to previous outcomes, noting whether or not there has been any change (improvement or decrease) in test outcomes in the appropriate assessment section of the report.
3. List all tests performed and the results obtained.

Ear Examination and Otoscopy

Audiologists perform the external ear examination and otoscopy in order to describe and identify, not diagnose abnormalities of the pinna, periauricular structures, ear canal, and tympanic membrane. When reporting ear examination results absent of apparent disorder, it is best to indicate that results are *unremarkable* rather than *normal*, because the latter term may fall within the confines of diagnosis.

1. Pinna and periauricular structures

   Note any malformations, growths, lesions (cuts or scabs) of or around the pinna, including the mastoid bone region.

2. Ear canal

   Document narrowing or obstructions of the ear canal (cerumen, excessive hair, foreign objects, growths); discharge (blood or other; describe consistency, e.g., color, thickness, etc.), or lesions along the canal wall.

3. Tympanic membrane

   Describe atypical findings such as clarity and color (cloudiness, redness, or yellowness), discharge, fluid bubbles, perforation, retraction, or bulging. Note the presence of a pressure-equalizing (PE) tube.

Pure Tone Audiometry

1. Describe the test technique used [e.g., standard audiometry, play, visual reinforcement audiometry (VRA), etc.]. If sound-field testing is conducted, results reflect the hearing of the better ear, if there is a difference. A rationale for using sound-field testing should be provided (e.g., child would not allow earphone placement), and earphone assessment should be attempted (and documented) in order to obtain ear-specific information. Indicate whether using a screening or diagnostic procedure.

2. The interpretation statement on hearing other than that which is normal should indicate the degree (amount), configuration (shape), and type (conductive, sensorineural, or mixed) of hearing loss for each ear if different, or indicate *bilaterally* if the hearing for both ears is the same (e.g., a moderate sloping to severe sensorineural hearing loss bilaterally). Categorize the degree of hearing loss as slight, mild, moderate, moderately-severe, severe, or profound. Note the configuration of hearing loss other than flat (e.g., rising, gradually or sharply sloping). If there is hearing loss in specific frequency regions, also report the range that is normal (e.g., normal hearing up to 1000 Hz sloping to a mild mixed hearing loss for the right ear). If the type of hearing loss differs within the same ear (i.e., conductive in the lower frequencies but sensorineural in the higher frequencies), specify each type rather than using the combined term *mixed*.

3. Indicate whether there is any asymmetry in pure tone findings between ears.

4. Report the two and three frequency pure tone averages (PTAs).

Speech Audiometry

1. Report the speech recognition thresholds (SRTs) and consistency with the two or three frequency PTAs.

2. Report the speech recognition scores (SRSs), the presentation levels used, and consistency of the SRS with the degree and

type of hearing loss. Classify the SRS as excellent, good, fair, poor, or very poor. Indicate if the SRS findings were poorer than expected or asymmetric between ears.

Immittance

1. Indicate whether using a screening or diagnostic procedure.
2. Note whether results of tympanometry, ipsilateral and/or contralateral acoustic reflex thresholds (ARTs), and acoustic reflex decay (ARD) are within normal limits, which is suggestive of normal middle ear functioning.
3. With tympanometric findings outside of normal range, describe aspects of the tympanogram such as peak admittance (abnormally low or high), middle ear pressure (excessively negative or positive), and ear canal volume (abnormally low or high) in addition to the classification (e.g., A, B, C), if used.
4. Ipsilateral or contralateral ARTs outside of normal range may be elevated or absent; specify frequencies tested; report results relative to the stimulus ear.
5. Classify ipsilateral or contralateral ARD as either positive or negative, and frequencies at which performed; report results relative to the stimulus ear.
6. Depending on the findings, indicate whether results are suggestive of a specific pathology. For example, reduced peak admittance, abnormally low ear canal volume, and absent ARTs would support impacted cerumen, particularly if observed on otoscopic examination. There is a fine line between *identifying* and *diagnosing* abnormality. Be careful to use phrasing of potential pathology in hypothetical rather than actual terms. For example, reduced peak admittance, excessively negative middle ear pressure, and absent ARTs coupled with otoscopic findings of redness of the tympanic membrane *may be suggestive of middle ear pathology such as otitis media*, but may not be stated as *indicating otitis media*. With PE tube placement, comment on function based on the ear canal volume reading. For example, an abnormally high ear canal volume reading would be suggestive of a patent (and normally functioning) PE tube. In the presence

of normal tympanometry and sensorineural hearing loss, ART and ARD outcomes may be interpreted to support either cochlear or retrocochlear pathology.

Behavioral Site-of-Lesion Tests

When site-of-lesion is of concern in patients with sensorineural hearing loss, several behavioral tests may be useful in providing further information to the standard audiometric battery in addition to electrophysiologic tests. Report findings from tone decay, short increment sensitivity index (SISI), or performance-intensity function for phonetically balanced (PI-PB) word tests as either positive or negative (the term *rollover* may be used with PI-PB outcomes). Indicate whether results support cochlear or retrocochlear pathology.

Electrophysiologic Tests

1. Report the purpose of the electrophysiologic test.
2. Indicate whether using a screening or diagnostic procedure.
3. In hearing estimation, ABR can be used to estimate hearing thresholds to a specific degree, frequency (with tonal ABRs), and type (with bone conduction ABR).
4. ABR conducted in neurologic assessment should be classified as normal or abnormal (which would be indicative of retrocochlear pathology).
5. Present otoacoustic emissions (OAEs) support normal cochlear outer hair cell function, whereas absent OAEs may suggest abnormal cochlear, outer, or middle ear disorder.
6. Vestibular function is assessed by tests such as (video-) electronystagmography (V/ENG), rotational chair, or posturography.

Clinical Impressions

Provide a summary of relevant findings. Do not present new information in this section, but refer to statements in prior assessment sections.

Recommendations

In cases where no significant hearing loss or other audiometric outcomes were noted, no further audiologic recommendations are
indicated. Further recommendations may include the following,
and should be indicated in order of importance:

1. Further testing
   a. Reevaluation to complete the hearing test, as is often
      required in pediatric populations
   b. Electrophysiologic tests (e.g., ABR, OAE, ENG)
   c. (Central) auditory processing tests

2. Follow-up testing
   a. To monitor hearing in patients with potential late-onset or
      progressive hearing loss, occupational or recreational
      noise exposure, or those taking ototoxic medications
   b. Following medical treatment
   c. Annual retesting

3. Rehabilitative options
   a. Amplification assessment, dispensing, verification, and
      follow-up of a new fitting
   b. Hearing aid checks for an existing fitting
   c. Cochlear implant evaluation

4. Hearing Conservation
   a. Use of hearing protection
   b. Monitoring use of ototoxic medication
   c. Counseling regarding hearing preservation

5. Referral to other professionals
   a. Speech-language pathologist
   b. Otologist or other medical specialist (i.e., pediatrician,
      general practitioner)
   c. Educational specialist
   d. Social worker
   e. Psychologist
   f. Genetic counselor

   Clinical interns
   (Names of students participating in evaluation)

Supervisor's name, degree, CCC-AuD

Audiologist

Institutional title (Professor, Clinical Supervisor)

Diagnostic Protocol Worksheet—Audiology

Client's Name   Date of Evaluation

History

Referral source

Informant

Informant reliability

Reason for concern

For a Child

Prenatal and birth history

Speech-language developmental milestones

Motor development milestones

For a Child or Adult

Medical history

Hearing history

Other evaluations

Prior and current therapies

Family history of hearing problems

Assessment Information

Behavioral observations

Reliability of testing

Changes from prior testing

Ear Examination and Otoscopy

Pinna and periauricular structures

Ear canal

Tympanic membrane

Pure Tone Audiometry

Test technique

Degree, configuration, type of hearing loss

Hearing asymmetry

Two and three frequency Pure Tone Averages PTAs

Speech Audiometry

Speech recognition threshold (SRT)

SRT consistency to PTA

Speech recognition score (SRS)

Presentation level of SRS

Consistency of SRS to pure tones

Immittance

Tympanometry

Ipsilateral, contralateral acoustic reflex thresholds (ARTs)

Acoustic reflex decay (ARD)

Behavioral Site-of-Lesion Tests

Tone decay

Short increment sensitivity index (SISI)

Performance-intensity function for phonetically balanced (PI-PB)

Electrophysiologic Tests

Auditory brainstem response (ABR)

Otoacoustic emissions (OAEs)

(Video) electronystagmography (V/ENG)

Rotational chair

Posturography

References

American Speech-Language-Hearing Association. (1996). *Central auditory processing: Current status of research and implications for clinical practice* (Technical Report). Rockville, MD: Author.

American Speech-Language-Hearing Association. (2005). *(Central) auditory processing disorders.* Rockville, MD: Author.

Brookshire, R. H. (1983). Subject description and generality of results in experiments with aphasic adults. *Journal of Speech and Hearing Disorders*, *48*, 342–346.

Carey, B. (2007). Bipolar soars as diagnosis for the young. *The New York Times*, September 4, A1; A15.

Council For Clinical Certification in Audiology and Speech-Language Pathology of the American Speech-Language-Hearing Association. (2007). 2007 Standards for the Certificate of Clinical Competence in Audiology, Revised July 2008. Retrieved February 28, 2009, from http://www.asha .org/about/membership-certification/certification/aud_standards_ new.htm

Damasio, H. (2008). Neural basis of language disorders. In R. Chapey (Ed.), *Language intervention strategies in aphasia and related neurogenic communication disorders* (5th ed., pp. 20–41). Baltimore: Lippincott Williams & Wilkins.

Goldfarb, R. (2006a). An atheoretical discipline. In R. Goldfarb (Ed.), *Ethics: A case study from fluency* (pp. 117–137). San Diego, CA: Plural.

Goldfarb, R. (2006). Differential diagnosis of adults with neurogenic communication disorders. In E. M. Walsh (Ed.), *Topics in Alzheimer's disease research* (pp. 90–108.). Hauppauge, NY: Nova.

Goldfarb, R., & Halpern, H. (1981). Word association of time-altered auditory and visual stimuli in aphasia. *Journal of Speech and Hearing Research, 24,* 234–247.

Martin, F. N., & Clark, J. G. (2009). *Introduction to audiology* (10th ed.). Boston: Allyn & Bacon.

Northern, J. (1995). *Hearing disorders* (3rd ed.). Boston: Allyn and Bacon.

Schiavetti, N., & Metz, D. E. (2006). *Evaluating research in speech-language pathology and audiology* (5th ed.). Boston: Allyn & Bacon.

Schuell, H. M. (1966). A re-evaluation of the short examination for aphasia. *Journal of Speech and Hearing Disorders, 31,* 137–147.

Schuell, H. M. (1973). *Differential diagnosis of aphasia with the Minnesota test* (2nd ed., revised by Sefer, J. W.). Minneapolis: University of Minnesota Press.

Schwartz, M. (1984). What the classical aphasia categories can't do for us, and why. *Brain and Language, 21,* 3–8.

Stach, B. A. (1998). *Clinical audiology: An introduction.* San Diego, CA: Singular.

St. Louis, K. O., & Myers, F. L. (2007). *Cluttering* (DVD No. 9700). Memphis, TN: Stuttering Foundation of America.

Weiss, D. (1964). *Cluttering.* Englewood Cliffs, NJ: Prentice-Hall.

Yaruss, J. S., LaSalle, L. R., & Conture, E. G. (1998). Evaluating stuttering in young children: Diagnostic data. *American Journal of Speech-Language Pathology, 7,* 62–76.

EXERCISES

I. Edit the Diagnostic Report: Speech-Language Pathology

Comment on items highlighted in bold and followed by a number in parentheses.

Speech-Language Evaluation

Name: Jane Jones

Address: 123 Articulation Road

Garden City, NY 11530

Telephone Number: 516-877-4777

Date of Evaluation: 7/19/08

Date of Birth: 1/15/1994

Chronological Age: **14.6** (1)

Background Information

Jane Jones is a **fourteen year old** (2,3) female who was evaluated at the Center for Communication Disorders. She was accompanied by her mother, who served as a reliable informant. Jane reportedly has no significant birth/medical history. Her mother reported that Jane suffered from frequent ear infections the first 2 years of her life. Tubes were not inserted because antibiotics always resolved the infection. Ms. Jones stated that Jane did not have any feeding or swallowing difficulties at any time.

Jane's developmental milestones were achieved at or before typical ages. She sat at 7 months, crawled at 8 months, walked at 11 months, and stood alone at 10 months of age. She babbled "very early," spoke her first words "early," and put 2 to 3 words together at 12 months. She spoke in sentences soon after her first birthday and was described as being "very verbal."

Ms. Jones reported that Jane has become more aware of a lisp within the last year. She is an active, friendly child who engages in basketball, track, and socializing with her friends. Jane said her trouble producing /s/ sounds does not bother her but other people are aware of it.

She (4) had speech therapy in 4th grade for 2 to 3 months, but no progress was seen. She was given exercises to do at home but they were not successful. Jane's father reportedly has a slight lisp but has never had speech therapy. She is entering high school in the fall and is motivated to improve articulation.

Assessment Information

A speech and language assessment was performed at the Center on July 19, 2008. Jane was cooperative throughout the evaluation. She had an appropriate attention span and was able to comprehend and complete all tasks given to her by the clinicians.

Formal Testing

The ***Goldman Fristoe II*** (5) *Test of Articulation* (GFTA-2) was used to evaluate Jane's speech production. The results from the GFTA-2 revealed an interdental lisp on **[s] and [z]** (6) phonemes in all positions of words and sentences.

Pragmatics

Jane's pragmatic skills were informally assessed throughout the evaluation. She demonstrated adequate conversational skills, as she was able to appropriately initiate, maintain, and terminate interactions with the clinicians. She appropriately used and maintained eye contact throughout the assessment when engaged in conversation.

Language Comprehension

Jane's language comprehension abilities were judged to be within functional limits, as she appropriately responded to questions asked by the clinicians. She was able to understand and follow instructions given by the clinicians and was able to maintain conversation.

Language Production

Formal language assessment was not performed because it was observed that Jane's expressive language abilities **are** (7) within functional limits. She demonstrated age-appropriate vocabulary and appropriate syntactic abilities. She was able to formulate complex sentences using correct grammatical morphemes and sentence structure.

Speech Production

Jane's articulation skills were assessed by the GFTA-2. Although she demonstrated an interdental lisp, her overall intelligibility was not affected. Her errors were typical of speakers who demonstrate an interdental lisp, as she produced the /θ/ for the /s/ and /ð/ for the /z/ phonemes in all word positions. However, Jane was stimulable for correct production of her error sounds.

Oral Facial Examination

An oral peripheral examination revealed **normal** (8) facial symmetry of the jaw, lips, and tongue. Tongue range of motion, lip closure, and diadochokinetic rate appeared to be within normal limits. Jane demonstrated good oral-nasal shifting and adequate closure of the velopharyngeal port. Jane exhibited a unilateral tongue thrust when performing a dry swallow. She was stimulable for reduction of tongue thrust via myofunctional therapy techniques.

Voice and Fluency

Perceptual judgments indicated vocal quality, resonance, **pitch, and loudness** (9) were typical for age and gender. Fluency was within normal limits.

Audition

On 7/19/08 Jane demonstrated hearing in both ears to be **within normal limits** (10). Both ears were tested at 20 dB HL at 1000 Hz, 2000 Hz, 3000 Hz, and 4000 Hz.

Clinical Impressions

Jane Jones presented with a mild interdental lisp. Her language production and comprehension skills appeared to be within functional limits. Jane's language skills, voice, fluency, and audition were all within normal limits. Jane would benefit from speech therapy focusing on her articulation errors.

Recommendations

Individual speech therapy is recommended once a week for 30 minutes. Initial goals of therapy should focus on:

1. Correct production of /s/ starting from the /t/ position; and
2. Eliminating or reducing the tongue thrust.

Hildred Schuell
Clinical Intern

Robert West, Ph.D., CCC-SLP
Speech-Language Pathologist
Clinical Supervisor

II. Edit the Diagnostic Report: Audiology

Comment on items highlighted in bold and followed by a number in parentheses.

Audiologic Evaluation

Name: Tyler Frank

Address: 9 Reade Road

Maintown, NY 12345

Telephone: (987) 654-3210

Date of Evaluation: 7/10/08

Date of Birth: 3/1/06

Chronological Age: 2:4

History

Tyler Frank, a 2:4-year-old male, was seen at the Center for Communication Disorders on July 10, 2008, for an initial audiological evaluation. He was referred for this evaluation by the County Early Intervention program to rule out hearing loss as a cause of his speech and language delay. **Mrs. Frank** (1) reported that Tyler has been receiving speech and language therapy **3** (2) times a week for about 6 months. According to Mrs. Frank, Tyler's motor milestones were **developed in the appropriate time frame** (3); however, his speech and language milestones were delayed. **Mrs. Frank** (4) indicated that there is no familial history of hearing loss. Medical history revealed that Tyler was hospitalized for a severe fever, **but other than that he did not suffer any pertinent** illnesses (5).

Assessment Information

Tyler was cooperative during the audiologic assessment.

Pure Tone Audiometry

Audiological test results obtained via **VRA** (6) in the sound field were considered to be of good reliability. Responses to warbled tones were obtained at **15 dB** (7) for the frequencies of **500–4k** Hz (8).

Speech Audiometry

A speech detection threshold in sound field was obtained at 20 dB HL.

Immittance

Acoustic immittance measures revealed Type A tympanograms bilaterally.

Clinical Impressions

Audiologic results revealed normal hearing in at least the better ear. Acoustic immittance measures indicated normal middle ear function bilaterally. Based upon these results, hearing loss may be ruled out as a contributing factor to Tyler's speech and language delay.

Recommendations

The results of the evaluation were discussed with Mrs. Frank, and **reevaluation** (9) in 6 months for **monaural thresholds** (10) was recommended.

Kelsy Masters
Clinical Intern

Sara Booth, Au.D., CCC-A
Audiologist
Clinical Supervisor

ANSWERS

Exercise I

1. Jane is 14½ years old, or 14.5; her age should be expressed as 14:6, not 14.6, to indicate 14 years, 6 months.

2. A number of 10 or more should be expressed as a numeral, not a word.

3. Hyphens are needed for "14-year-old."

4. Use a noun, rather than a pronoun (which might refer to Jane or her mother in the present example), at the beginning of a paragraph.

5. Be consistent in use of Roman numerals versus Arabic numbers.

6. Indicate phonemes with slash marks, e.g., /s/ and /z/, not brackets.

7. Keep tenses consistent.

8. In most cases, use the word *typical*, rather than *normal*.

9. The terms *pitch* and *loudness* are used correctly here, because they are psychological phenomena. If the clinician used acoustic instrumentation, then the correct terms would be *frequency* and *intensity*.

10. It is appropriate to use the term *normal* in the context of "within normal limits."

Exercise II

1. Specify who Mrs. Frank is; most likely she is Tyler's mother, but without clarification the reader may also assume she is Tyler's grandmother.

2. Numbers less than 10 should be expressed as a word, not a numeral.

3. The phrase can be simplified by stating that the "developmental motor milestones were appropriate."

4. There is excessive reference to Mrs. Frank. The sentence can be reworded without referring to her again: "There was no reported history of familial hearing loss."

5. The wording is awkward; a better way to phrase this would be, "however, no other significant history was noted."

6. Always define an abbreviation the first time it appears in the report, no matter how common the usage: "visual reinforcement audiometry (VRA)."

7. The decibel (dB) unit must always be referenced; in this case it is dB HL. Note the space between dB and HL.

8. The unit kilohertz (kHz) is equal to 1000 Hz; note that the small letter *k* does not follow the number. In this example there is inconsistency with the usage of the units in the frequency range, which should be written as either .5–4 kHz or 500–4000 Hz.

9. Specify that a *hearing* reevaluation is being recommended.

10. The phrasing is incorrect; it should be stated "in order to obtain monaural hearing thresholds."

CHAPTER 8

Clinical Reports and Referrals

The diagnostic report (see Chapter 7) is the most comprehensive account of professional interaction with a patient. Often the diagnostic report is sent to other professionals as part of the referral process and may be accompanied by a cover letter along with copies of clinical assessment outcomes, such as an audiogram or speech documents that may be sent. However, the lengthy diagnostic report may not be the appropriate reporting format to document information for all clinical services or practice sites. In this chapter other clinical report formats will be discussed and presented, in addition to considerations in the correspondence and sharing of written information with other professionals.

Informed Consent and Permission

Justification

Prior to initiating therapy, a speech-language pathologist or audiologist, or the institution that employs them, should obtain a signed informed consent from the consumer of therapeutic services. If the consumer is a minor child or a disabled adult, an adult advocate should provide informed consent. The form specifies terms of treatment and permission for release of information. The clinician should also obtain permission to make audio-visual recordings for therapeutic and educational purposes and permission to use instrumentation and edibles. Where appropriate, as in a medical or educational setting, there should also be permission to permit observation of therapy and diagnostic sessions. Where HIPAA regulations prevail (see Chapter 3, Ethics of Professional Writing), confidentiality of individually identifiable health information must be assured. The following informed consent form, based on the one used at Adelphi University, may be modified to suit the needs of other institutions or individual practitioners.

Informed Consent Form

I consent and request that the following service(s) be performed for (circle)

myself   my spouse   my child   _____

(print name)

at the Center for Communication Disorders at State University (check services requested):

_____ Speech-Language Evaluation

_____ Speech-Language Therapy

_____ Audiological Evaluation

_____ Hearing Aid Evaluation

_____ Other Services (specify): _____

I understand and agree to the following:

a. Services will be performed by or under the supervision of an appropriately licensed and certified speech-language pathologist or audiologist;
b. Graduate and undergraduate student interns may participate in the delivery of any and all services;
c. Promises for success of treatment cannot be made;
d. All information will be kept confidential unless written consent to release information is obtained from me;
e. If authorization for services has been denied by my insurance company, I will be responsible for all charges incurred;

   f. If the Center for Communication Disorders is not a participating provider for my insurance company, I will be
responsible for all charges incurred;

   g. I give permission for the Center for Communication
Disorders to release information required to receive
approval and reimbursement for services to the source of
reimbursement for such services (e.g., insurance company,
Early Intervention Program, school district, etc.).

Please send me a copy of any Evaluation or Progress Report relating
to the above services.

Print Name _____   Sign Name _____

Relationship to Client _____   Date _____

Primary Insurance _____   Secondary Insurance _____

Permission Form

I understand and agree to the following:

   a. In order to execute certain therapeutic and diagnostic
procedures, it is occasionally necessary to use instruments,
such as a penlight or tongue depressor, or edibles, such as
crackers or juice, in the course of treatment or evaluation.
Before using any edible item, the clinician will consult with
me to ensure that there are no contraindications, such as
allergies, to the use of that item.

   b. I consent to the use of any instrument or material within
the scope of practice for use by the speech-language pathologist or audiologist in order to conduct effective assessment
and treatment.

   c. I agree to permit students enrolled in pertinent academic
coursework, trainees, or clinical fellows to participate in the
evaluation and/or treatment procedures, which will be
conducted under the supervision of an appropriately
licensed and certified professional.

   d. I consent to the use of audio-visual recordings for therapeutic, educational, and research purposes.

Please list any contraindications, such as allergies or other medical conditions, to the use of edibles: _____

Print Client's Name _____

Signature (Client, Parent, or Advocate) _____

Relationship to Client _____ Date _____

Types of Professional Reports

Treatment Plan

Include long- and short-term goals, as in the following example:

1. *Long-Term Goals of Therapy*
   a. AB will demonstrate improved pragmatic/social interaction skills.
   b. AB will improve receptive language skills.
   c. AB will improve expressive language skills.

2. *Short-Term Goals of Therapy*
   a. AB will maintain purposeful eye contact for 3 to 5 seconds during 16/20 consecutive conversational exchanges for three consecutive sessions.
   b. AB will follow two-step directives 16/20 times for three consecutive sessions.
   c. AB will produce transitive verbs in a Picture Exchange Communication System (PECS) 16/20 times in three consecutive sessions.

Progress Report

Review long- and short-term goals and provide results, as in the following example:

1. The first goal was to have AB demonstrate improved pragmatic/social interaction skills. Tasks included establishing and maintaining trunk alignment while seated, establishing eye contact for 3 to 5 seconds during conversational

exchanges, and making appropriate transitions from one task to another. AB achieved criterion of 80% correct for 20 trials over three consecutive sessions in these tasks. However, she continued sporadic tantrums in transitions between activities, and required verbal and visual prompts to establish and maintain eye contact.

2. The second goal was for AB to improve receptive language skills. Tasks included having AB identify pictures of common objects, independently point to pictures of verbs (e.g., *want*), and respond to two-step directives during activities. With the use of PECS, AB achieved criterion of 80% correct for 20 trials over three consecutive sessions in pointing to pictures of nouns and verbs and in following two-step directives.

3. The third goal was for AB to improve expressive language skills. Tasks included labeling action verbs, independently initiating a conversational exchange expressed vocally or with PECS, and independently using PECS for the purpose of requesting. Using PECS, AB met criterion of 80% correct for 20 trials over three consecutive sessions for labeling transitive but not intransitive verbs; for independently initiating a conversational exchange; and for requesting action, but not for requesting information or clarification.

Guidelines for Writing Progress Reports in Speech-Language Pathology

PROGRESS REPORT

Date

Client

Address

Telephone

Date of Birth

Age

Frequency/Length of Therapy Sessions (individual and group therapy)

Clinician

Supervisor

<u>PRESENTING PROBLEM</u>
(All section headings should be all capital letters and underlined.)

This is a historical overview of the client's communication problem. In the first paragraph, provide a brief description of the presenting problem, including the nature of the communication impairment and initial severity rating. You may find this information in the initial evaluation report. In the second paragraph, summarize therapy history and progress to the beginning of the current semester.

<u>GOALS OF THERAPY</u>

Present the information in a list format or in narrative form. Include the semester goals, not the short-term objectives, taken from your treatment plan.

<u>TEST DATA</u>

Include updated test results performed during the current semester.

<u>PROCEDURES AND PROGRESS</u>

Address each short-term goal with a paragraph of text. Procedures include materials, activities, and, most importantly, therapeutic techniques, such as the types of prompts and cues used to facilitate success. When reporting progress, do not overload this section with numbers reflecting percentages of accuracy in individual therapy sessions, but rather try to describe what the client is or is not able to do.

<u>PRESENT STATUS</u>

Briefly note the client's strengths and weaknesses. Highlight areas that need to be addressed in future therapy.

<u>RECOMMENDATIONS</u>

Include such recommendations as:

1. cessation or continuation of therapy,
2. number and length of sessions per week,

3. individual or group treatment,
4. future therapy goals,
5. referrals, and
6. suggestions for home practice.

Clinician's Name   Supervisor's Name and Credentials

Clinical Intern   Title

Progress Report: Writing Style Worksheet

1. Use the client's complete name.
2. Write age in years and months for clients under age 18, and years only for those older than 18. Remember to use a colon, not a decimal point, between years and months (e.g., 5 years, 9 months is 5:9, not 5.9).
3. Avoid ambiguous terms and colloquialisms. For example, always use a referent, rather than a pronoun, such as *she* or *that*, for the first notation in a paragraph. Be specific: "The clinician used stickers to get the client to say something," should be rewritten as, "The clinician used stickers to motivate the client to use the auxiliary verbs, *is*, *are*, and *am*."
4. Use language that can be understood by the reader. Define all technical terms and professional language, give examples for clarification, and use the phrase, *characterized by*, after a diagnostic label.
5. Use specific, accurate, brief sentences. Avoid verbosity and jargon.
6. Use complete verb forms; avoid contractions and hyphens.
7. Use active rather than passive verbs. Avoid such qualifiers as *somewhat*, *quite*, and *very*.
8. Write in the third person rather than the first person. Refer to yourself as *the clinician*, not as *I* or *me*.
9. Follow the rules for use of numerals described in Chapter 1. In general, use words to express one through nine and numerals for 10 and above. However, as noted in the numeral expressed as *Chapter 1* above, there are exceptions to the rule.
10. Express behavioral data mathematically, where possible. When reporting progress, include the number of trials to

criterion and number of consecutive sessions in addition to the percent correct. Writing *80% correct responses* can mean 4 of 5 correct or 8 million out of 10 million. In general, collect data for at least 20 trials over three consecutive sessions before reporting the percent correct. In cases where performance is variable, use such quantifiers as *some* or *most*. Indicate whether criterion levels were reached for your clinical goals.

11. Use operational definitions and operationally written goals. These are statements of observed behavior that the client exhibits as a result of your clinical intervention strategies. Avoid such mentalistic terms as *learn*, *understand*, and *know*, and use operational terms such as *categorize*, *retell*, or *repeat*.

12. Do not refer to *lesson plans* when you mean *clinical intervention strategies*, or to *teaching* when you are *testing clinical hypotheses*. Our jobs would be much easier if we could, for example, eliminate word retrieval impairments by teaching vocabulary lessons.

Edited Progress Report in Speech-Language Pathology

The progress report below, with identifying information changed, includes comments in brackets that relate to information highlighted in boldface type and indicated by the left arrow. In general, there is a good deal of useful information in the progress report, but it is compromised by imprecise and overly verbose writing, or *flabby prose*. Before searching the Internet for the South Beach Writing Diet, please note some of the specific comments.

Date: August 9, 2008   Client: Hillary Bloomingdale

Address: 1000 Third Avenue,
          New York, NY 10065

Telephone: (212) 794-0000   Date of Birth: 7/23/35   Age: 73

Frequency/Length of therapy sessions:

     Individual: 1×/wk for 45 minutes

     Group: 1×/wk for 60 minutes

Clinician: Barack McCain

Supervisor: **Dr. Robert Goldfarb, PHD**, CCC-SLP ← [writing Dr. and PhD (not *PHD*) is redundant]

PRESENTING PROBLEM

Mrs. Bloomingdale ← [form of address, e.g., *Mrs.* or *Ms.* is established by the institution] is a **73 year old woman** ← [need hyphens for *73-year-old*] who presents with mixed (flaccid, spastic) dysarthria resulting from cerebral hemorrhage in 2004. The client's speech is poorly intelligible and can be **characterized by** breathiness, hypernasality, poor breath support, consistent articulation errors, slow rate, strain-strangled voice quality, and poor variety in pitch and volume ← [good expansion of *characterized by*]. Saliva management is a cause of concern to the patient, as she is constantly wiping her mouth with a handkerchief and apologizing for the presence of extra saliva. The client has reported a hiatal hernia, which manifests **itself** ← [delete—redundant] in **gastoesophagael** ← [two spelling errors in *gastroesophageal*] reflux disease, causing pain and heartburn. The client currently receives physical therapy for **right sided** ← [add hyphen] weakness as a result of the stroke. Cognition is intact, and Mrs. Bloomingdale presents **herself** ← [delete—redundant] as a bright, sophisticated, and **highly opinionated** ← [wrong word—it means *stubborn*; also delete modifier] woman.

Mrs. Bloomingdale has attended both group and individual therapy regularly since May 2007. She appears to be **highly** ← [delete modifier] motivated and **utilizes** ← [*Uses* is preferred here and almost everywhere.] the strategies **taught** ← [*Established* is a better word, as therapy involves testing clinical hypotheses, and does not follow a curriculum.] during therapy in order to be understood by the listener. Despite the requirement that the speaker put forth considerable effort in understanding Mrs. Bloomingdale, **she** ← [referent is unclear] is determined to be understood and uses **many different modalities** ← [Specify whether the modalities are auditory, visual, graphic, etc.] to reach **intelligibility** ← [should be *comprehensibility* as context is involved]. During previous semesters, the client was **taught** ← [*trained*] to tap out each syllable with her finger and increase her vocal intensity to improve **intelligibility** ← [*Intelligibility*, based on an acoustic measure, is used correctly here]. She is currently working on improving her articulation, prosody, and vocal quality.

GOALS OF THERAPY

1. Mrs. Bloomingdale will improve her **prosody skills** ←[use the adjective, *prosodic*, to modify the noun, *skills*] by using correct intonation and stress patterns.
2. Mrs. Bloomingdale will use **the** ← [delete] proper breath support during speech.

> Goals 1 and 2 do not have measurable objectives.

3. Mrs. Bloomingdale will **improve** her articulation of /s/ using the auditory discrimination and phonetic placement approaches. ← [Set a criterion for improvement, based on a percentage derived by dividing number of correct responses by number of trials, and maintained over a specified number of therapy sessions.]
4. Mrs. Bloomingdale will **incorporate her speaking strategies** while conversing with peers. ← [This is too general to be a useful goal.]

TEST DATA

No standardized tests were performed during the current semester.

PROCEDURES AND PROGRESS

Authors' note: Only the first goal is analyzed for writing.

1. Mrs. Bloomingdale will improve her prosodic skills by using correct intonation and stress patterns.

A method called *shadowing* was used to improve prosody and increase the naturalness of the client's speech. The clinician read a **passage** ← [add comma] and the client was instructed to repeat **after the clinician** ← [delete—redundant] and follow her stress and intonation patterns. While shadowing the clinician, Mrs. Bloomingdale's speech sounded less **robotic**. ← [Use a more behavioral descriptor.] In addition to shadowing, the clinician **also** ← [Delete as redundant, because the sentence started with *in addition*.] presented the client with written questions with arrows indicating **proper** ← [Use a behavioral descriptor, e.g., *rising* or *falling*.] intonation and had the client read them aloud. Mrs. Bloomingdale had **difficulty managing pitch changes** ← [Use a behavioral descriptor.] **in her voice** ← [delete as redundant] as **appose** ← [misspelled *opposed*] to pitch. **An exercise was done where** ← [delete] the clinician said a sentence while raising either the volume or **pitch** ← [use *frequency* to correspond with *volume*] **of her voice** ← [delete phrase, but insert comma] and Mrs. Bloomingdale was asked to identify which aspect was changed. The client's motivation and cooperation facilitated improvement in her prosodic skills. However, **much work** ← [therapy] is still needed **in order** ← [delete] to **further** ← [delete] increase the naturalness of the client's speech.

Audiogram Form Report

In settings where audiologic assessment procedures, findings, and terminology are well understood, it is common to use an abbreviated reporting form instead of the comprehensive diagnostic report format. The client's actual audiogram (in expanded form) may serve as the report itself (Figure 8–1). The audiogram report includes graphic or tabular information of clinical outcomes (e.g., pure tones, speech audiometry, immittance), in addition to a written summary section (Stach, 1998). The audiogram form report is commonly used in the exchange of information with audiologists, otologists, and hearing aid dispensers, and is often the reporting format used in the patient charts of hospital or medical settings. The brevity of this type of report form creates the advantage of reducing time in both the recording and reading of information in the often fast-paced health setting.

Medical Chart Logs/Reports

A typical reporting format used in hospitals or medical-based clinics or centers is the medical chart log or report. The writing of logs or reports in medical charts is extremely brief and includes only the most pertinent information, characterized by the use of standard abbreviations (see Chapter 1, Getting Started, and sample list below), short phrases, or fragmented sentences. This writing style meets the need of quick documentation and reading of information for professionals in facilities where many patients are seen in short time blocks (Bickley & Hoekelman, 1999; Seidel, Ball, Dains, & Benedict,

Audiology Center

Name _____ Age _____ Date _____

Audiologist _____ Audiometer _____

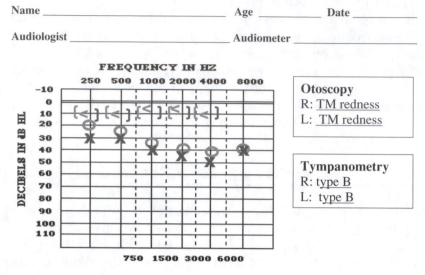

Otoscopy
R: <u>TM redness</u>
L: <u>TM redness</u>

Tympanometry
R: <u>type B</u>
L: <u>type B</u>

Speech Audiometry

	SRT dB HL	SRS %	SRS dB HL
R	30	100	65
L	30	96	65

HISTORY:
<u>failed hearing screening</u>

RESULTS:
<u>Otoscopy: redness of tympanic membranes (TM) bilaterally</u>
<u>Pure Tones: mild to moderate conductive hearing loss bilaterally</u>
<u>Immittance: type B patterns bilaterally</u>

RECOMMENDATIONS:
1. <u>medical referral to assess middle ear status</u>
2. <u>re-test post medical treatment or follow-up</u>

Figure 8–1. Sample audiogram report.

2003). Although appropriate to the health or medical facility, a more formal reporting format (see prior sections in this chapter) may be necessary when sending reports to other professionals. In audiology, it is common practice to use the audiogram report form (see above) as the medical chart entry.

Common medical chart abbreviations are used in communication sciences and disorders. For a more complete list of abbreviations in our discipline, see Chapter 1.

abs	absent
AD	right ear
ART	acoustic reflex threshold
AS	left ear
AU	bilaterally
c/o	complains of
CHL	conductive hearing loss
CAE	complete audiologic evaluation
CR	correct responses
DOB	date of birth
Dx	diagnosis
ENT	ear, nose, throat
FH	family history
F/U	follow-up
Hx	history
NA	no answer; not applicable
OM	otitis media
OME	otitis media with effusion
PECS	Picture Exchange Communication System
Pt	patient
Rec	recommendation

s	without
sec	seconds
SNHL	sensorineural hearing loss
Sx	symptoms
T & A	tonsillectomy and adenoidectomy
TM	tympanic membrane
URI	upper respiratory infection
WNL	within normal limits

Example of a Medical Chart Report: Speech-Language Pathology

Log Note: 9/10/08

Maintain eye gaze 3–5 sec: 18/20 CR = 90%

Transition to task: 4/5 CR = 80% (one tantrum)

Label verbs in PECS task: 10 consecutive "I want"

Point to Boardmaker nouns: 14/20 CR = 70% (used "pizza" as default choice)

Example of a Medical Chart Report: Audiology

Evaluation: 9/10/08

F/U CAE 13 yo = TM redness AU; Mild to moderate CHL AU; type B tymps AU; abs ARTs AU

Rec: 1. ENT 2. retest

Expanded Version:

A complete audiologic evaluation follow-up was conducted on this 13 year-old patient.

Otoscopy: redness of the tympanic membranes bilaterally

Pure Tones: Mild to moderate conductive hearing loss bilaterally

Immittance: Type B patterns bilaterally; absent contralateral middle ear reflexes

Recommendations:

1. Medical referral to assess middle ear status
2. Retest post-medical follow-up or treatment

Professional Correspondence

Correspondence often takes the form of a request for information from an outside agency or professional, referral for additional service, or compliance with a request for information or service.

Professional Referrals/Sending Reports

Often the proper clinical care of a patient requires further assessment or treatment by other professionals in communication disorders or those in other disciplines (e.g., medical, educational, psychological). Patients may be referred to you as the communication disorders specialist, or you may be making the referral. In either case, an exchange of information regarding the patient will be required.

Following the regulations of the Health Insurance Portability and Accountability Act (HIPAA) of 1996, it is imperative that a signed release of information form be obtained from the client or legal guardian prior to providing any information, oral or written, to other individuals including professionals who may be involved with the client's case. A signed release is necessary even if a report is to be sent to the professional who may have referred the client to you in the first place. It is important to recognize a patient's right to refuse disclosure of information.

Letters to Professionals

Letters to other professionals may be written for the purposes of information request, referral, or gratitude, and may also serve as a cover letter accompanied by an additional report or copies of clinical outcomes regarding a patient. Depending on the nature of the professional relationship, a formal cover letter usually accompanies a written report of information that is sent to other professionals. The formality of a cover letter may be omitted when corresponding with a professional with whom one is very familiar. It may not be conventional practice in some settings, where briefer reporting practices are preferred (see sections on report forms above).

There are two variations of letter formats in the reporting of patient information in professional correspondence: one in which a separate cover precedes the formal report, and the other where the report is written in a letter format.

Cover Letter Format

Sender Contact Information

> Address
>
> Telephone Number
>
> E-mail Address

Date

Recipient Contact Information

> Recipient Name
>
> Title
>
> Address

Salutation

Begin this section with "Dear (title and name):" making sure to use the correct title (e.g., Dr., Ms., Mr.) and spelling of the first and last names. Use a proper salutation even when sending an e-mail; do not begin with the informal greeting of "Hi."

Body of the letter

The first sentence should begin with a statement of the purpose of the correspondence, such as for referral, reporting, or request of information on a specific patient. Identify the patient and the type, location, and date of the service conducted or requested, as applicable. If clinical findings are to be communicated, the next sentences should refer to the report and whether it is attached as a hard or electronic copy. In the letter report format (see example below), the report itself may be embedded into the letter in subsequent paragraphs. The last sentences in the body of the letter may thank the recipient for a request of information, and add or refer to your listed contact information.

Closing

End the letter with a cordial term such as "Sincerely," "Respectfully," or "Yours truly."

Name and Signature

Type your name with degree and certification credentials, and place your handwritten signature just above it. For e-mail transmission, provide an electronic signature.

Example Cover Letter for Speech-Language Pathology Report

Note that date, signature, and paragraphs are indented.

Speak the Speech
1501 Hamlet Street
Stratford, CT 12345
1-800-SCENEII

September 24, 2008

Sara Booth, AuD, CCC-A
I'm All Ears
321 Blastoff Street
Cape Kennedy, FL 10987-6543

Dear Dr. Booth:

I am referring AB for a complete audiological evaluation. She failed a pure tone hearing screening bilaterally for the frequencies 500, 1000, 2000, and 4000 Hz at 20 dB HL. Enclosed please find a copy of her speech and language evaluation.

If you need additional information, please do not hesitate to contact me.

Yours truly,
Anne Hathaway, MS, CCC-SLP
Speech-Language Pathologist

Example Cover Letter for Audiology Report

Note that date, signature, and paragraphs are all flush with the left margin. Both indented and flush styles are acceptable in a cover letter.

Center for Communication Disorders
Jamestown, NY 98765

September 10, 2008
Andrew House, MD
723 Main Avenue
Jamestown, NY 98765

Dear Dr. House:

I am referring Susan Shore, age 13 years, for middle ear evaluation. She was referred to the Center for Communication Disorders for a complete audiologic assessment as a result of failing a hearing screening in school. Audiologic and immittance findings are consistent with middle ear pathology.

Enclosed please find a copy of the audiologic report, audiogram, and immittance findings. Pending any medical treatment, a hearing retest is recommended. Please contact me should you require any further information.

Sincerely,
Sara Booth, AuD, CCC-A
Audiologist

Example Letter Report: Audiology

Center for Communication Disorders
Jamestown, NY

September 11, 2008

Dear Dr. House:

I am referring Susan Shore, age 13 years, for middle ear evaluation. She was referred to the Center for Communication Disorders for a complete audiologic assessment as a result of failing a hearing screening in school. Audiologic and immittance findings were obtained on September 10, 2008, and are as follows:

AUDIOLOGIC ASSESSMENT

Otoscopy
Redness of the tympanic membranes was noted bilaterally.

Pure Tone Audiometry
Mild to moderate conductive hearing loss bilaterally.

Speech Audiometry
Speech recognition thresholds (SRTs) are consistent with pure tone findings. Speech recognition scores (SRSs) are excellent.

Immittance
Type B patterns bilaterally with absent contralateral acoustic middle ear reflexes, consistent with middle ear pathology.

CLINICAL IMPRESSIONS

Clinical findings of tympanic membrane redness, conductive hearing loss, and type B tympanograms with absent middle ear reflexes are consistent with middle ear pathology.

RECOMMENDATIONS

1. Medical evaluation to assess middle ear status.
2. Retest post medical treatment or follow-up.

Sincerely,
Sara Booth, AuD, CCC-A
Audiologist

Correspondence via Electronic Media

Present-day professional correspondence involves interaction via hard copy ("snail mail"), telephone, or electronic media. Increasingly, delayed or instant text-messaging through telephone or computer media has become a popular electronic communication form in average daily interaction. Similarly, electronic communication of patient records through facsimile (fax) or Internet transmission is commonly used in professional correspondence. Reports may be scanned or sent as text documents in e-mail attachments, or faxed from original hard copies to the recipient. Facsimiles may also be the legal equivalent of an original document, which should be familiar to those of us who have served on jury duty.

Irrespective of transmission form, proper professional correspondence etiquette requires some formal introductory commentary to precede the electronic submission. The "cover letter" in electronic correspondence may follow a formal cover letter style (see section above) or a less formal style of a few lines of text (under the heading, say, of "Fax Transmission Sheet") that would include a salutation, reference to an attached or sent document regarding the specific patient, and a closing.

Certainly, all forms of electronic communication, even the less formal, should follow proper professional writing style, form, and content. This applies to any type of professional communication, even the nonclinical. For students, this would include electronic correspondence with professors or clinical supervisors in the academic setting. E-mails from students without proper formal salutation, or with use of the colloquial *hey*, may be perceived as rude, whereas errors in spelling or grammar from prospective students may leave the impression of someone incapable of graduate-level work. A simple rule of thumb would be to follow and apply the principles of professional writing in *any* type of professional interaction.

References

Bickley, L. S., & Hoekelman, R. A. (1999). *Bates' guide to physical examination and history taking* (7th ed.). Philadelphia: Lippincott Williams & Wilkins.

Health Insurance Portability and Accountability Act (HIPPA) of 1996, Public Law 104-191, 104th Congress.

Seidel, H. M., Ball, J. W., Dains, J. E., & Benedict, G. W. (2003). *Mosby's guide to physical examination* (5th ed.). St. Louis, MO: Mosby.

Stach, B.A. (1998). *Clinical audiology.* San Diego, CA: Singular.

EXERCISES

1. Informed consent is needed:
   a. only if the consumer is a minor child or a disabled adult
   b. to permit HIPAA regulations to prevail
   c. to assure confidentiality of individually identifiable health information
   d. before the clinician uses edible items in therapy
   e. to permit the clinician or institution to charge fees for services

2. "AB will maintain purposeful eye contact for 3 to 5 seconds during 16/20 consecutive conversational exchanges for three consecutive sessions" is an example of a:
   a. long-term goal
   b. short-term goal
   c. treatment plan
   d. progress report
   e. status report

3. In a progress report, the *presenting problem* includes:
   a. the historical overview of the client's communication problem
   b. the goals of therapy
   c. test data
   d. procedures
   e. recommendations

4. The problem with writing, "The clinician used stickers to get the client to say something," is that it includes:
   a. passive rather than active verbs
   b. use of the first person rather than the third person
   c. verbosity and jargon
   d. language that cannot be understood by the reader
   e. ambiguous terms

5. The abbreviation OME refers to:
    a. organic mental evidence
    b. other means of expression
    c. otitis media with effusion
    d. one more example
    e. outer middle ear

ANSWERS

1. The correct answer is *d*. It is important to determine if there are medical conditions, such as diabetes or allergies, that may impact choice of edibles. Any consumer (not only those identified in *a*) should provide informed consent. HIPAA regulations (*b*) are federal law, and supersede local informed consent. Assurance of confidentiality for individually identifiable health information (*c*) is the guiding principle of HIPAA, and does not require the consumer's consent. A policy to require payment for services rendered (*e*) is not contingent on informed consent, although the consumer may sign a statement accepting responsibility for charges not covered by insurance.

2. The correct answer is *b*. Note that there are measurable behavioral goals, including number of trials to criterion. A long-term goal (*a*) relating to eye-gaze behavior might be "AB will demonstrate improved pragmatic/social interaction skills." A treatment plan (*c*) includes both long-term and short-term goals. A progress report (*d*) includes the results of clinical intervention, not the plan, and progress is written in the past tense, not the future tense. A status report (*e*) is written in the present tense, not the future tense.

3. The correct answer is *a*. Indicate the type and severity of the problem at intake. Short-term and long-term goals of therapy (*b*) are taken from the treatment plan. Test data (*c*) may form the basis for identifying the type and severity of the communication disorder, but should be included in a separate section. Procedures (*d*) include materials, activities, and therapeutic techniques. Recommendations (*e*) come at the end of the report, whereas the presenting problem comes at the beginning.

4. The correct answer is *e*. The clinician used stickers to motivate the client to say the auxiliary verbs *is*, *are*, and *am*, not merely to "say something." Choice *a* is not correct, because the statement was written in the active voice (as compared to this sentence, written in the passive voice).

Choice *b* is not correct, because a construction using the first person would be, "I used stickers to . . . " Verbosity and jargon (*c*) would include using "adhesive-backed reinforcement stimuli to elicit production of functors." The preceding sentence might also qualify as *d*.

5. The correct answer is *c*. We're just playing with our language toy in the other examples.

CHAPTER 9

Writing for Professional Advancement

There are a number of written documents essential for advancement as students in academic programs and for securing employment as future professionals in communication sciences and disorders. This chapter will focus on those documents.

Resumes

The resume (*resumé*, *résumé*; French meaning *summary*) is intended to be a brief (one- to two-page) written synopsis of an individual's educational background, skills, and experience. In essence it can be thought of as a large business card. A more detailed, lengthier version known as the *curriculum vitae* (*CV*; Latin meaning *course of life*) is commonly used in academic, legal, and scientific settings (Friedman, 2007). Typically, the student and future professional in communication sciences and disorders will be using the resume format, unless hired by a college, university, or research institution, for which the CV is appropriate.

Although the most common purpose of the resume is for gaining employment, it may also be useful to the student in providing information for the preparation of letters of recommendation, applications for service or leadership positions, awards, or scholarships. The resume is a work in progress throughout one's career; the information should continually be updated to reflect the latest academic or professional developments. As such, the resume also serves as a record of one's academic and professional achievements and experiences. Students should therefore begin to develop their resumes early on during their program of study, adding and modifying the information as it changes during the course of academic and professional life. A good suggestion would be to make modifications as they occur rather than when the resume is needed. This will prevent lapses in memory of specific details and allow easy access to an already updated resume at a moment's notice.

The main purpose of the resume when job searching is to get noticed and land an interview. In writing the resume, particularly for purposes of employment, certainly clarity and style are important, but brevity is of the essence. Unlike the CV, which can go on for pages with detailed information, the resume is meant to capture important details confined to no more than two (but preferably one) pages of space. Employers or personnel reviewers frequently must get through dozens of resumes before deciding which candidates to interview, and often do so by a quick overview of the information. Indeed, a study suggests that only 1 minute or less is spent by most hiring reviewers in reading a resume and forming an impression on an applicant's qualifications, with preferences shown for organized, conventional-style resumes (Helwig, 1985). It is therefore in the applicant's best interest to follow a basic guide for resume preparation, as described below (McDaniels, 1990; O'Hair, Friedrich, Wiemann, & Wiemann, 1997; Rosenberg & Hizer, 1990; Seiler & Beall, 1999).

Although there is no standard resume style to which you must adhere, the most commonly used is the *chronological* format, which uses headings to group items listed, with the most recent first (i.e., in reverse chronological order). The order and specific titles may differ and should be tailored to the individual, but typical headings of information following the letterhead would include education, certifications/licenses, professional experience, awards/honors, publications, professional presentations, research, professional affiliations/activities, skills, and references. Adding a section on *objectives* is optional, but really unnecessary in our very specialized professions as the listed degrees, certifications, and skills will clarify the targeted position. In addition, stating an objective on the resume that is too narrow might limit job opportunities. For example, if a prospective job seeker indicates an objective of hearing aid fitting and dispensing, an employer of a multiservice site who is seeking someone to conduct hearing evaluations and amplification services may bypass this applicant. Statements of purpose usually belong in the cover letter (see section below).

There are numerous professional Web-based programs and for-hire assistive services for resume preparation, but most universities offer tips (in-person or via the Internet) to students for free. It is strongly recommended that the student take advantage of these academic services but independently lay out and type the resume on a personal computer, making sure to save it on both hard and soft drives. Because the resume will be repeatedly updated, one must be able to access the information quickly and easily; this will prevent the need to start from square one each time a resume is needed.

Following are *do's* and *don'ts* tips with a basic resume layout to assist with creating a high-quality resume.

Do's

1. Above all, be truthful! A resume, as any written professional document, is bound by ethical reporting.
2. Distinguish headings by using distinctive typeface such as uppercase or bolding; separate items under each heading by using dates, titles, or bullets, making sure to be consistent throughout. Omit headings that don't apply, or add ones that may be more appropriate.
3. List all items under headings in reverse chronological order; use the present tense for current activities and past tense for previous ones.
4. Use a minimum 11 or 12 point type and standard (e.g., Times New Roman, Arial) font (larger type may be used for headings); smaller fonts may be difficult to read and fancy fonts may transform into indecipherable characters in e-mail transmission.
5. Print the resume on letter size, heavy weight (22–25 lb.) cotton-fiber content, light-colored paper using margins no more than 1 inch left and right and no less than ½ inch top and bottom.
6. If the resume is sent by e-mail as an attachment, confirm that it was received and that it could be opened and was legible for the recipient.

Don'ts

1. Don't include a photograph.
2. Don't include such personal information as social security number, date of birth, military status, marital status, or number of children.
3. Don't puff up the resume with excess verbiage or irrelevant information. A sincere, parsimonious, and focused resume is usually received as well as or better than one that runs on for many more pages.
4. Don't create a resume with "bells and whistles." A too-busy, colorful, or atypical resume style may give the impression of immaturity or lack of seriousness.

Letterhead

The letterhead (appears without the heading) is typically centered at the top of the document with your name (in bold uppercase letters) and contact information, including address, telephone number (if multiple numbers, designate home number vs. cell), and e-mail address.

Education

List the most current degree first, ending with the baccalaureate degree. You need not list your high school education. Include the name of the institution, city and state where the degree was awarded, the degree and field of study (major and minor areas), and year of completion. If the degree is in progress, indicate the date it will be conferred. List degree honors (e.g., Summa or Magna Cum Laude); inclusion of a grade point average (GPA) is optional, but should definitely be omitted if less than a 3.0.

Certifications/Licenses

List the dates and titles of any professional or related certifications or licenses received.

Professional Experience

This is probably the most important section of the resume and the one a reviewer will look at first. In reverse chronological order, list the dates of employment, job title, employer, city, and state. For students just graduating, it is fine to list practica experiences; just modify the heading to indicate this. Don't include experiences outside the field of communication sciences and disorders, such as part-time jobs undertaken while a student. However, individuals who have had important positions in other fields and have changed careers may use the section on employment history to show evidence of leadership and responsibility that should be highlighted. Importantly, you want to be able to support your experience or skill in specific areas by stating the job responsibilities and tasks executed. This can be conveyed by using action verbs such as *conducted*, *evaluated*, or *performed* rather than passive words such as *assisted*, *observed*, or *participated*. Separate items using a bulleted list format.

Awards/Honors

List the titles and dates of the specific award, scholarship, or designated honor (e.g., dean's list). Separate the headings and respective items when substantive.

Publications

List publications in reverse chronological order, similar to APA-style referencing (see Chapter 5, Using Library Resources), indicating whether journal articles were published in refereed or nonrefereed periodicals (designated subheadings may be used if substantive).

Professional Presentations

Follow APA-style referencing (see Chapter 5, Using Library Resources) to list each presentation, the type of session (e.g., paper, poster), and whether the professional meeting is national, state, or regional.

Research

Use this section to indicate the participation in or conduct of research-related activities such as those related to doctoral or masters theses, independent study, or research assistantships.

Professional Affiliations/Activities

Indicate memberships or offices held in professional organizations. Include the dates, position (e.g., member, officer), and title of the organization. Title the heading as *Affiliations* or *Activities* for listing nonprofessional campus or community organizations or volunteer affiliations.

Skills

Highlight special skills such as fluency in a foreign language or American Sign Language.

References

References may be listed as "provided on request" or may include names, titles, and contact information for at least three individuals who have agreed to provide a reference.

Figures 9–1 and 9–2 are sample resumes for a hypothetical student of speech-language pathology or audiology. More examples on resumes can easily be found using an Internet search.

Cover Letters for Resumes

Appropriate employment-seeking etiquette requires that a cover letter precede the resume. Whereas the resume is a uniform, universal document to be sent to many individuals, the cover letter must be tailored to fit the contact name, site of employment, job title, and responsibilities of the targeted position. Because the cover letter is usually a first point of contact with a prospective employer, it will provide a first impression of you, and in this case, first impressions do matter.

JOHN Q. PUBLIC
1000 Third Avenue
New York, NY 10065
(212) 794-1000
jqp@bloomingdales.com

EDUCATION
Adelphi University, Garden City, NY
M.S. in Speech-Language Pathology, Phi Delta Kappa, 2008
Queens College, CUNY, Flushing, NY
B.A. in Linguistics and Communication Disorders, 2006

INTERNSHIPS
Peninsula Medical Center, Far Rockaway, NY
Speech-Language Pathology Intern, February 2008–May 2008
  Conducted bedside swallowing evaluations
  Evaluated videofluoroscopic examinations
  Provided speech-language therapy to adults with swallowing disorders

Herbert G. Birch School, Flushing, NY
Speech-Language Pathology Intern, September 2007–December 2007
  Evaluated preschool children for speech and language
  Provided speech-language therapy to preschool children

Hy Weinberg Center for Communication Disorders, Garden City, NY
Speech-Language Pathology Intern, September 2006–May 2007
  Provided individual speech-language therapy to preschool children,
    and group language stimulation to preschool children in TOTalk
  Provided individual and group therapy to adults with aphasia

AWARDS/HONORS
AAC Institute Award, ASHA Division 12, 2007

PROFESSIONAL AFFILIATIONS/ACTIVITIES
Student Member, National Student Speech-Language-Hearing
Association, 2006–2008
Student Volunteer, New York State Speech, Hearing, and Language
Association Convention, April 2008

SKILLS
American Sign Language, Level 4

REFERENCES
Available upon request

Figure 9–1. Resume Example for Speech-Language Pathology

JANE DOE

123 Fourth Lane
Maintown, NY
(012) 345-6789
jdoe@doe.com

EDUCATION
Long Island Doctor of Audiology (AuD) Consortium
Adelphi University, Hofstra University, and St. John's University, NY
Doctor of Audiology (AuD), to be conferred May 31, 2009
Adelphi University, Garden City, NY
B.A. in Communication Sciences and Disorders, Magna Cum Laude, 2004

INTERNSHIP EXPERIENCE
Long Island Medical Center, New Hyde Park, NY
Audiology Student Intern, January 2008–present
    Perform hearing aid evaluations on pediatric and adult populations
    Dispense hearing aids

Island Hearing Screening Program, Jericho, NY
Audiology Student Intern, September 2007– December 2007
    Performed hearing and outer and middle ear screenings on pediatric
        clients
    Tabulated screening data

Hy Weinberg Center for Communication Disorders, Garden City, NY
Audiology Student Intern, September 2006–May 2007
    Conducted hearing evaluations on pediatric, adult, and geriatric clients
    Completed (Central) Auditory Processing Evaluations
    Evaluated hearing aid function using electroacoustic analysis, real ear

AWARDS/HONORS
Adelphi University Student Leadership Award, 2007

PROFESSIONAL AFFILIATIONS/ACTIVITIES
Student Member, American Academy of Audiology, 2004–2008
Student Volunteer, Annual Conference of the American Academy of
Audiology, April 2008

SKILLS
Fluent in Spanish

REFERENCES
Available upon request

Figure 9–2. Resume Example for Audiology

Keep the cover letter formal by using professional language and using proper rules of writing and spelling, similar to writing a proper letter. It is wise to be concise, limiting the length to one page. A hard-copy cover letter should be printed on good-quality paper, similar to the resume. Although it is acceptable to send cover letters via e-mail, a professional formality must be maintained.

Following is a description of the cover letter format and a sample.

Resume Cover Letter Format

Sender Contact Information

Address

Telephone Number

E-mail Address

This section can alternatively be added at the bottom of the letter, or incorporated into the ending paragraph.

Date

Recipient Contact Information

Recipient Name

Title

Address

Salutation

Begin this section with "Dear (title and name):" making sure to use the correct title (e.g., Dr., Ms., Mr.) and spelling of the first and last names. If unsure, it is best to use a general salutation (e.g., "To the Reviewing Committee:"). Use a proper salutation even when sending an e-mail; do not begin with the informal greeting of "Hi."

Beginning Paragraph

The first paragraph should begin by expressing interest in the position, detailing why you are interested, and indicating the name of the person who referred you, if applicable.

Middle Paragraph

The second and subsequent paragraphs should indicate, briefly, your experience and why you would be appropriate for the job. Indicate any other pertinent information such as unique qualifications.

Final Paragraph

End the letter by thanking the recipient for consideration of your application, and indicate when and how you will follow up. It is particularly important that you follow up (after 1 week is appropriate) because letters do get lost in the mail and e-mails may not open. Add or refer to your listed contact information as well in case the employer wishes to contact you.

Closing

End the letter with a cordial term such as "Sincerely," "Respectfully," or something similar.

Name and Signature

Type your name with degree and certification credentials, and place your handwritten signature just above it. For e-mail transmission, provide an electronic signature.

Sample Resume Cover Letter

Jane Doe
123 Fourth Lane
Maintown, NY
(012) 345-6789
jdoe@doe.com

May 1, 2009
Ellen Smith, PhD
Best Hearing Care, Inc.
567 Eighth Drive
Maintown, NY 12345

Dear Dr. Smith:

I am writing to express my interest in the clinical audiology position available at your center. I will be receiving my doctoral degree in audiology (AuD) from the Long Island Doctor of Audiology Program, New York, on May 31, 2009. My advisor, Prof. Yula Serpanos, suggested I contact you regarding this position.

I noted in the job description that you are seeking experience with diagnostic hearing evaluation and amplification fitting in pediatric populations. In my 4 years of academic and clinical training including my current internship at the Long Island Medical Center, I have acquired knowledge and skill in these areas and feel that I am well prepared and qualified for clinical work in this capacity. Please see the attached resume for more complete information on my education and training. A hard copy of both this letter and my resume will be following.

I thank you for your consideration of my application. I will be in touch next week in order to obtain more information. You may contact me if you wish at the phone and e-mail address listing above. I look forward to speaking with you soon.

Sincerely,

Jane Doe

Jane Doe

Portfolios

The portfolio, a selection of one's representative academic or professional work and accomplishments, has gained popularity for use in both academia and job searching in many professions, including communication sciences and disorders. The collection of documents comprising the portfolio is housed either electronically or in bound hard copy. In academic programs, students may be required to maintain a *developmental portfolio*, or one that serves the purpose of documenting a student's progress in the mastery of the required knowledge and skill areas. Upon graduation, a *career portfolio* may be maintained for professional use in order to maintain a record of professional development and achievements.

Similar to the resume, the portfolio is a work in progress throughout one's academic or professional career, where materials can be updated as changes occur. A hard-copy portfolio can be compiled in a three-ring binder, and materials can easily be added or removed as needed. The hard-copy career portfolio can be taken to an interview where the reviewer can peruse the documents on site. It is wise to keep a second hard-copy of the items in the portfolio and to save the items electronically. Though electronic portfolios have the advantage of saving space and items into memory, hard copies provide easier viewing of numerous pages and may be preferred by most reviewers; a diskette of the portfolio can then easily be provided if requested. Following is a suggested list of items to include in a professional portfolio as applicable (McLaughlin et al., 1998; Poore, 2001; Straub, 1997).

1. Academic transcript (only for a student applying for a first job)
2. Resume
3. Copies of degrees, licenses, certificates, attendance at relevant professional workshops
4. Samples of clinical evaluations, projects, reports (see below for specific clinical samples in speech-language pathology or audiology)
5. Professional presentations
6. Performance reviews
7. Student evaluations of teaching, clinical supervision
8. Recommendation letters
9. Reference list

Portfolio Checklist of Clinical Work in Audiology

Standard Audiologic Evaluation

☐ Child

☐ Adult

Behavioral Pediatric Testing

☐ BOA

☐ VRA

☐ Play Audiometry

Behavioral Hearing Screening

☐ Child

☐ Adult

Outer/Middle Ear Screening

- ☐ Child
- ☐ Adult

Behavioral SOL Testing-Adult

- ☐ ABLB
- ☐ MLB
- ☐ PI-PB: Standard
- ☐ PI-PB: Modified (Abbreviated)
- ☐ SISI: Standard
- ☐ SISI: High Intensity
- ☐ Tone Decay: Carhart
- ☐ Tone Decay: Olsen/Noffsinger

Functional Testing

- ☐ Stenger test
- ☐ Stenger procedure for hearing estimation

(Central) Auditory Processing Screening

- ☐ Child
- ☐ Adult

(Central) Auditory Processing Evaluation

- ☐ Child
- ☐ Adult

Earmold Impression

- ☐ Child
- ☐ Adult

Hearing Aid Selection/Fitting

☐ Electroacoustic analysis

☐ Real ear analysis: Child

☐ Real ear analysis: Adult

ABR-Adult

☐ Click-evoked (SOL)

☐ Tonal (hearing estimation)

ABR-Child

☐ Click-evoked (SOL)

☐ Tonal (hearing estimation)

☐ Screening

OAE-Adult

☐ DPOAE diagnostic

☐ DPOAE screening

☐ TEOAE diagnostic

☐ TEOAE screening

OAE-Child

☐ DPOAE diagnostic

☐ DPOAE screening

☐ TEOAE diagnostic

☐ TEOAE screening

Vestibular Assessment

☐ ENG

☐ Rotational Chair Test

☐ Posturography

Calibration

☐ Audiometer

☐ Soundfield

Portfolio Checklist of Clinical Work in Speech-Language Pathology (Adelphi University Codes)

The portfolio is a developmental scrapbook of evidence of meeting ASHA's standards. Page protectors and dividers provide for ease of reviewing. Maintain this archive electronically in order to provide a CD portfolio. Scan in graded rubrics when using a digital portfolio. See portfolio checksheet for specific contents.

The first page should be the checksheet followed by your most recent transcript and then the KASA form completed as of that date (Table 9-1, Table 9-2, Table 9-3, and Table 9-4).

The portfolio should include three client studies: one child, one adult, and one culturally-linguistically diverse. Include a client study from student teaching, if appropriate, as well as one from a diagnostics practicum.

The client study must include the treatment plan, one session plan (with rationales for goals and procedures), a reflection on that session (how you did and how the client did), the progress note, and a reflection at the end of the semester on that client.

1. *Demonstrating Competency.* Use the KASA form (see Table 9-1 through Table 9-4) to maintain this record of how well you are mastering material. Simultaneously, the instructor is documenting the same. If you feel you need additional experience in any area, please consult with your advisor.
2. *Remediation Plans.* In the event you do not meet the minimum standard in a particular competency area (e.g., you fail an exam or get a poor score on a rubric in class or therapy), you must meet with the instructor to devise a remediation plan. Your grade will not change for that assessment. However, at the end of the semester, the instructor will determine whether you have successfully demonstrated competency in that area or whether additional demonstration is necessary.

Table 9–1. Sample Documentation for Articulation

	Knowledge				Assessment Skills				Intervention Skills			
	Evidence type	Rating/ grade	Instructor	Date	Evidence type	Rating/ grade	Instructor	Date	Evidence type	Rating/ grade	Instructor	Date
Articulation 610	Course grade	A	Lederer	F07	Midterm phono process analysis	45/50	Lederer	F07	Final therapy presenta-tion	34/40	Lederer	F07
611	Course grade	A–	Redstone	F07	Video analysis	19/20	Redstone	F07	Client study	42/50	Redstone	F07
Clinical					666 Goldman-Fristoe	N/A	Montano	SS 08	N/A			
Clinical					N/A				Self-reflection: client with dysarthria	Satis-factory	Goldfarb	Sp 08

Table 9–2. Knowledge and Skills Documentation

	Knowledge of Disorder (III-C)				Assessment Knowledge/Skills (III-D; IV-F; IV-G)				Intervention Knowledge/Skills (III-D; IV-F, IV-G)			
	Evidence type	Rating/ grade	Instructor	Date	Evidence type	Rating/ grade	Instructor	Date	Evidence type	Rating/ grade	Instructor	Date
Articulation 610	Course grade											
611	Course grade											
Clinical												
Clinical												
Fluency 620	Course grade											
Clinical												
Clinical												
Voice 630 (611)	Course grade											
Clinical												
Clinical												

continues

Table 9–2. *continued*

	Knowledge of Disorder (III-C)				Assessment Knowledge/Skills (III-D; IV-F; IV-G)				Intervention Knowledge/Skills (III-D; IV-F, IV-G)			
	Evidence type	Rating/ grade	Instructor	Date	Evidence type	Rating/ grade	Instructor	Date	Evidence type	Rating/ grade	Instructor	Date
Language 603	Course grade											
638	Course grade											
634	Course grade											
Clinical												
Clinical												
Hearing 606	Course grade											
Clinical (other than 668)												

	Knowledge of Disorder (III-C)				Assessment Knowledge/Skills (III-D; IV-F; IV-G)				Intervention Knowledge/Skills (III-D; IV-F, IV-G)			
	Evidence type	Rating/ grade	Instructor	Date	Evidence type	Rating/ grade	Instructor	Date	Evidence type	Rating/ grade	Instructor	Date
Swallowing 646	Course grade											
636	Course grade											
Clinical												
Clinical												
Cognitive Linguistic 624	Course grade											
Clinical					At least one client study (treatment plan, session plan, progress note, self-reflection)	1-2-3			At least one adult client	1-2-3		
Clinical												

continues

Table 9–2. *continued*

	Knowledge of Disorder (III-C)				Assessment Knowledge/Skills (III-D; IV-F; IV-G)				Intervention Knowledge/Skills (III-D; IV-F; IV-G)			
	Evidence type	Rating/ grade	Instructor	Date	Evidence type	Rating/ grade	Instructor	Date	Evidence type	Rating/ grade	Instructor	Date
Social-behavioral 673	Course grade											
Clinical												
Other												
Modalities (AAC) 672	Course grade											
Clinical												
Clinical												
Screening/ Prevention 666					Speech-language screening	1-2-3						
668					Hearing screens	668 Grade =						
634												
Other												

228

Table 9–3. Additional Knowledge Assessments

	Evidence Type	Grade/Rating	Instructor	Date
Basic sciences (III-A): 1 Bio, 1 Phys sci; 1 Math; 1 Social Science	Transcript			
Human Comm Sciences (III-B): prerequisites 600	Transcript			
613	Course grade			
	Course grade			
Department policies and Procedures (III-H)	Grad manual			
Ethical Conduct (III-E) 648	Code of ethics sign-off			
670 (NIH Certification)				
Other				

continues

229

Table 9–3. *continued*

	Evidence Type	Grade/Rating	Instructor	Date
Research and Evidence-Based Practice(III-F) 670 660	Course grade EBP project			
Contemporary Professional Issues (III-G) 648 Other	Position statement activity sign off			
Certification, specialty recognition, licensure, TSSLD, graduation requirements, Praxis, comps (III-H)	Graduation seminar materials			

Table 9–4. Additional Skills Assessments

Evidence Type	Grade/Rating	Instructor	Date
Oral language (IV-B) Screening by advisor	Pass or Fail? If fail, results of diagnostic Therapy?		
Written language (IV-B) 648 Critical observation	1-2-3		
Clinical writing (IV-B) 660 Lesson plans; tx plans; progress notes	Mean score from all final supervisor evals		
666 Diagnostic reports	Score from final eval		
Interaction with professionals and families, collaboration, ethics, professional behaviors, counseling (IV-G3) Supervisor evals	S/NI/U		
648			
660			
661/674 or 662	S/NI/U		

continues

231

Table 9-4. *continued*

	Evidence Type	Grade/Rating	Instructor	Date
Delivering services to CLD populations (IV-F; IV-G)	At least one client study (treatment plan, session plan, progress note, self-reflection, client reflection)	1-2-3		
Other (e.g., 603 or 638 paper)				
Self-evaluation of practice 648	Essay	S/NI/U		
660	Essay	S/NI/U		
661/674	Essay	S/NI/U		
662	Essay	S/NI/U		
400 hours (IV-C, IV-D: 25 observation & 375 direct; 150 TSSLD)				
Summative Assessment (V-B)	COMPS	Pass or Fail?		
Exit survey (submit to office)				

U = Unsatisfactory   NI = Needs improvement   S = Satisfactory

3. *Clinical Practica*

    SPH 648: First in-house (Hy Weinberg Center)

    SPH 660: Second in-house (Hy Weinberg Center)

    SPH 661 or SPH 674/675: Externship or Clinical Practice in a School

    SPH 662: Externship (all take)

    SPH 666: Diagnostics practicum

    SPH 668: Audiology practicum

For All CSD Students:

- ☐ ASHA Knowledge and Skills Assessment (KASA) maintained by you

- ☐ Clinical Seminar critical observation and scored rubric

- ☐ Clinical Practicum Internship
    - ☐ One client study (treatment plan, one session plan with reflection of therapy, progress note, single subject research, or evidence-based practice project)
    - ☐ All supervisor evaluations
    - ☐ Knowledge, skills, dispositions self-evaluation

- ☐ One graded paper or project dealing with cultural diversity in SLP

- ☐ One graded paper or project dealing with technology

- ☐ Other individual graded papers or projects, such as narrative analysis, therapy plan, augmentative project, clinical case study, parent education materials

- ☐ Comprehensive examination

- ☐ Final self-evaluation

- ☐ Praxis report, if taken prior to graduation

For Candidates Seeking Initial Certification as Teacher of Students with Speech and Language Disabilities

- ☐ School observation, interview, and rubric

- ☐ LAST and ATS-W scores

- ☐ Clinical Practice in a School Setting/Bilingual School Setting
  - ☐ One client study, including IEP, session plan with reflection, progress note
  - ☐ One diagnostic report
  - ☐ Cooperating teacher evaluations
  - ☐ University supervisor evaluations

For All Other Candidates, Including TSSLD Holders or Non-Teacher Track Students

- ☐ Clinical Practicum Externship
  - ☐ One client study, including IFSP, IEP, or treatment plan, and a session plan with reflection
  - ☐ One diagnostic report
  - ☐ Supervisor evaluations
  - ☐ Self-reflection

For All Candidates: Additional Recommended Artifacts

- ☐ Evidence from volunteer work or unique experiences

- ☐ Your resume

- ☐ Letters of recommendation

Multiple-Choice Tests

Students take multiple-choice tests from elementary through graduate school, often from instructors who have had little or no formal training in preparing them. Professionals may write these questions as part of student assessment in a course, or in clinical practice for assessing reading comprehension or higher cognitive functions.

A multiple-choice item is an objective test question containing alternative response choices. The introductory statement, called the *stem*, presents the situation, poses the problem, and/or asks the question. Each question usually has four or five *options*, or possible responses to a question. The *key* is the option that is the correct answer. The other options are called *distractors* or decoys, which should be plausible but incorrect choices.

The Stem

Examinees often complain that the stem is so lengthy and ambiguous that the test item requires separating the wheat from the chaff more than revealing knowledge and skills. The sentence structure of a stem should be clear and direct. The stem should include all information necessary for the examinee to understand the intent of the item, but should not provide clues that will make it easy to detect the key. Rather than having words or phrases repeated in all of the options, they should appear once in the stem. Typical stems use the format of a direct question or an incomplete statement. A stem should avoid the format of filling in a blank, for example, *To evaluate communicative responsibility in stuttering, _____ should be avoided*, because the examinee needs to look back and forth between the stem and the options to try out the choices. Also, a multiple-choice item should not be a disguised true-false question, as in, *Which of the following statements about play therapy is true?*

The Options

The key, or the correct option, must be unequivocally correct, and the distractors indisputably wrong. Distractors or decoys should attract examinees who do not have adequate knowledge and skill, and not those who are confused by such terms as *all of the above except for C*. Although the authors enjoy a pun as much as anyone, examinees can be thrown by a bizarre or humorous decoy. Accordingly, the *levator linguini* should not be listed as a possible muscle of the tongue.

Applicants for ASHA's Certificate of Clinical Competence must achieve a score of 600 out of a range of 250 to 990 on the Praxis II

Table 9–5. Speech-Language Pathology Praxis Examination Content Categories: Scores in Speech-Language Pathology from 9/1/05 to 8/31/06 (N = 6,872)

Test Category	National Points Available Range	Average Performance Range
I. Basic Human Communication Processes	20–21	9–13
II. Phonological and Language Disorders	19–23	13–16
III. Speech Disorders	14–17	9–12
IV. Neurogenic Disorders	21–22	13–17
V. Audiology/Hearing	6–7	N/A
VI. Clinical Management	20–23	13–18
VII. Professional Issues/ Psychometrics/Research	9–12	6–8

Examination, which is a multiple-choice test (Table 9–5 and Table 9–6). The same exam is used by many states in the United States as one of the criteria for awarding licensure as a speech-language pathologist or audiologist. Whereas it is not the intention of the present authors to give specific test-preparation strategies to readers, it seems appropriate to present something of a guide to how multiple-choice items are written.

The Praxis Examination includes three types of questions, grouped according to cognitive levels, or the mental processes required in the problem-solving situation.

Level I questions assess knowledge, requiring the cognitive behavior of remembering and understanding previously learned information. There are relatively few Level I questions on the Praxis, because they require memorization rather than application of the knowledge in professional practice.

Examples of Level I questions follow.

Table 9–6. Audiology Praxis Examination Content Categories

Content Categories	Approximate Number of Questions	Approximate Percentage of Examination
I. Basic Human Communication Processes	31	26%
II. Prevention/Identification	12	10%
III. Behavioral Assessment/ Interpretation	16	13%
IV. Electrophysiological Measurement/Interpretation	10	8%
V. Rehabilitative Assessment	13	11%
VI. Rehabilitative Technology	13	11%
VII. Rehabilitative Management	13	11%
VIII. Professional Issues, Psychometrics, Research	12	10%

Note: Available at http://www.ets.org/Media/Tests/PRAXIS/pdf/0340.pdf

SLP Example

> The external or superior laryngeal nerve, a branch of Cranial Nerve X, the vagus, innervates which of the following intrinsic muscles of the larynx?
>
> A. posterior cricoarytenoid
> B. *cricothyroid*
> C. lateral cricoarytenoid
> D. transverse arytenoid
> E. thyroarytenoid

Selecting the correct answer of *B* requires only that the examinee recall its innervation, although it might be helpful to recall that all the other intrinsic laryngeal muscles are innervated by the recurrent laryngeal nerve. The question does not require application or interpretation, which might be addressed by a question regarding the effect of impaired innervation to cricothyroid on vocal pitch.

Audiology Example

> The ASHA 2005 air conduction pure tone guideline
> *minimally* requires testing of the following frequencies:
>
> A. 500, 1000, 2000 Hz
> B. 250, 500, 1000, 2000, 4000 Hz
> C. 250, 500, 1000, 2000, 4000, 8000 Hz
> D. *250, 500, 1000, 2000, 3000, 4000, 6000, 8000 Hz*
> E. 250, 500, 750, 1000, 1500, 2000, 3000, 4000, 6000,
>   8000 Hz

In selection of the correct answer *D*, the examinee is required to recall the specific pure tone frequencies that should be tested, but is not asked to indicate procedures related to hearing assessment.

Level II questions assess basic knowledge in context, requiring the cognitive behavior of interpretation, or understanding the *why* and *how* of a situation. The question might present a problem that can be solved by understanding a theory, principle, or technique.
    Examples of Level II questions follow.

SLP Example

> Aphasia syndromes represent an aphasia type at only
> one arbitrary point in time, but aphasia is a migratory
> disorder. Which migration might happen in aphasia?
>
> A. Broca's to Wernicke's to anomic
> B. *Jargon to conduction to anomic*
> C. Transcortical motor to global to Broca's
> D. Anomic to Wernicke's to jargon
> E. Transcortical sensory to Broca's to anomic

Selecting the correct answer of *B* requires that the examinee apply theories and patterns of recovery in aphasia, specifically regarding type and severity of the disorder. Aphasias cannot migrate from fluent to nonfluent or vice versa (A, E), nor can they migrate from less impaired to more impaired (C, D).

Audiology Example

> This auditory pathway is responsible for sound inhibition:
>
> A. *efferent*
> B. afferent

C. ipsilateral
D. bilateral
E. bone conduction

Choosing the correct option *A* requires an understanding of and ability to differentiate among different aspects of auditory function (i.e., afferent vs. efferent sound pathways, bone conduction hearing) and sound presentation (ipsilateral, contralateral).

Level III questions assess evaluation and decision making, requiring the cognitive behavior of synthesis of elements into a comprehensive whole. The questions often include hypothetical case information, and simulate the process of designing or modifying treatment based on evidence.

Examples of Level III questions follow.

SLP Example

Which of the following impairments may occur in traumatic brain injury (TBI), but not in aphasia?

A. poor word retrieval
B. poor reading and writing
C. semantic and phonemic paraphasias
D. circumlocutions
E. *disproportionately impaired pragmatic skills*

Selecting the correct answer of *E* requires that the examinee understand clinical characteristics of language impairments in aphasia and TBI, and synthesize the principle that individuals with aphasia communicate better than they speak, whereas the reverse is true for individuals with language and communication impairments secondary to TBI.

Audiology Example

A patient with a mild conductive hearing loss will likely exhibit a speech recognition threshold (SRT) of _____:

A. 0 dB HL
B. 10 dB HL
C. *30 dB HL*
D. 60 dB HL
E. 80 dB HL

In choosing option *C* the examinee must know the decibel levels that define a mild degree of hearing loss (26–40 dB HL), and know that the SRT is closely related to pure tone thresholds.

References

Friedman, J. P. (Ed.). (2007). *Dictionary of business terms* (4th ed.). Hauppauge, NY: Barron's Business Guides.

Helwig, A. A. (1985, December). Corporate recruiter preferences for three resume styles. *The Vocational Guidance Quarterly,* (34), 99–105.

McDaniels, C. (1990). *Developing a professional vita or resume.* Garrett Park, MD: Garrett Park Press.

McLaughlin, M., Vogt, M. E., Anderson, J. A., Dumez, J., Peter, M. G., & Hunter, A. (1998). *Portfolio models: Reflections across the teaching profession.* Norwood, MA: Christopher-Gordon.

O'Hair, D., Friedrich, G. W., Wiemann, J. M., & Wiemann, M. O. (1997). *Competent communication* (2nd ed.). New York: St. Martin's Press.

Poore, C. A. (2001). *Building your career portfolio.* Franklin Lakes, NJ: Career Press.

Rosenberg, A. D., & Hizer, D. (1990). *The resume handbook: How to write outstanding resumes and cover letters for every situation* (3rd ed.). Holbrook, MA: Adams Media Corp.

Seiler, W. J., & Beall, M. L. (1999). *Communication: Making connections* (4th ed.). Boston: Allyn and Bacon.

Straub, C. (1997). *Creating your skills portfolio: Show your accomplishments.* Menlo Park, CA: Crisp.

Index